Aging

Fight It
with
the Blood
Type Diet*

Also by Dr. Peter J. D'Adamo with Catherine Whitney

Eat Right 4 Your Type: The Individualized Diet Solution to Staying Healthy, Living Longer, and Achieving Your Ideal Weight

Cook Right 4 Your Type: The Practical Kitchen Companion to Eat Right 4 Your Type

Live Right 4 Your Type: The Individualized Prescription for Maximizing Health, Metabolism, and Vitality in Every Stage of Your Life

Eat Right 4 Your Baby: The Individualized Guide to Fertility and Maximum Health During Pregnancy, Nursing, and Your Baby's First Year

Eat Right 4 Your Type Complete Blood Type Encyclopedia

Blood Type O: Food, Beverage and Supplement Lists

Blood Type A: Food, Beverage and Supplement Lists

Blood Type B: Food, Beverage and Supplement Lists

Blood Type AB: Food, Beverage and Supplement Lists

Dr. Peter J. D'Adamo's Eat Right 4 (for) Your Type Health Library

Allergies: Fight Them with the Blood Type Diet®

Arthritis: Fight It with the Blood Type Diet®

Cancer: Fight It with the Blood Type Diet®

Cardiovascular Disease: Fight It with the Blood Type Diet®

Diabetes: Fight It with the Blood Type Diet®

Fatigue: Fight It with the Blood Type Diet®

Menopause: Manage Its Symptoms with the Blood Type Diet®

DR. PETER J. D'ADAMO
WITH CATHERINE WHITNEY

Dr. Peter J. D'Adamo's
Eat Right for Your Type
Health Library

Aging

Fight It
with
the Blood
Type Diet®

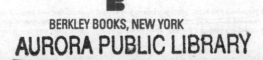

BERKLEY BOOKS, NEW YORK

THE BERKLEY PUBLISHING GROUP
Published by the Penguin Group
Penguin Group (USA) Inc.
375 Hudson Street, New York, New York 10014, USA
Penguin Group (Canada), 90 Eglinton Avenue East, Suite 700, Toronto, Ontario M4P 2Y3, Canada
(a division of Pearson Penguin Canada Inc.)
Penguin Books Ltd., 80 Strand, London, WC2R 0RL, England
Penguin Group Ireland, 25 St. Stephen's Green, Dublin 2, Ireland (a division of Penguin Books Ltd.)
Penguin Group (Australia), 250 Camberwell Road, Camberwell, Victoria 3124, Australia
(a division of Pearson Australia Group Pty. Ltd.)
Penguin Books India Pvt. Ltd., 11 Community Centre, Panchsheel Park, New Delhi—110 017, India
Penguin Group (NZ), Cnr. Airborne and Rosedale Roads, Albany, Auckland 1310, New Zealand
(a division of Pearson New Zealand Ltd.)
Penguin Books (South Africa) (Pty.) Ltd., 24 Sturdee Avenue, Rosebank, Johannesburg 2196,
South Africa

Penguin Books Ltd., Registered Offices: 80 Strand, London WC2R 0RL, England

While the authors have made every effort to provide accurate telephone numbers and Internet addresses at the time of publication, neither the publisher nor the authors assume any responsibility for errors, or for changes that occur after publication. Further, the publisher does not have any control over and does not assume any responsibility for author or third-party websites or their content.

AGING: FIGHT IT WITH THE BLOOD TYPE DIET®

A Berkley Book / published by arrangement with Hoop-A-Joop, LLC

PRINTING HISTORY
G. P. Putnam's Sons hardcover edition / January 2006
Berkley trade paperback edition / December 2006
Berkley mass-market edition / January 2007

Copyright © 2006 by Hoop-A-Joop, LLC
Blood Type Diet is a registered trademark owned by Peter J. D'Adamo
Cover design © 2006 by Thomas Tafuri
Cover photograph of Dr. D'Adamo © 2004 Martha Mosko D'Adamo

ISBN 978-0-425-21341-4

BERKLEY®
Berkley Books are published by The Berkley Publishing Group,
a division of Penguin Group (USA) Inc.,
375 Hudson Street, New York, New York 10014.
BERKLEY is a registered trademark of Penguin Group (USA) Inc.
The "B" design is a trademark belonging to Penguin Group (USA) Inc.

PRINTED IN THE UNITED STATES OF AMERICA

10 9 8 7 6 5

DEDICATED TO THE PIONEERING
BABY BOOMERS, HITTING SIXTY
IN 2006, WHO HAVE HERALDED
IN THE ERA OF HEALTHY,
HAPPY, VITAL AGING

Acknowledgments

THIS BOOK OFFERS THE BEST THAT NATUROPATHIC medicine and blood type science have to offer in helping people retain youthful well-being long into their lives. It has been a collaborative process, and I want to express my deep thanks to the people who have been involved in its creation.

I am most grateful to Martha Mosko D'Adamo, not only my partner in life and in parenting but also my partner in bringing the valuable wisdom about blood type to the world. Martha daily provides love, support, insight, and inspiration to all of my endeavors.

Catherine Whitney, my writer, and her partner, Paul Krafin, are invaluable word masters who have brought style and substance to the work.

My literary agent and friend, Janis Vallely, always takes time to listen and advise. Her quiet guidance and personal support make the work possible.

I would also like to acknowledge Laura Mittman, N.D., of the Institute for Human Individuality, who has been such a big help in my efforts to educate other professionals about the value of the Blood Type Diet.

Amy Hertz, my former editor at Riverhead/Putnam, was the force behind the blood type books. Denise Silvestro continues to shepherd the work with dedication and skill. Catherine's agent, Jane Dystel, contributes her ideas and support.

As always, I am extremely grateful to the wonderful staffs at Riverhead Books and Putnam. They have been tireless and enthusiastic, and their efforts have made it possible to continue bringing this important work to the world.

PETER J. D'ADAMO, N.D.

Contents

INTRODUCTION:
NEW TOOLS TO FIGHT AGING   I

WHY BLOOD TYPE MATTERS   4

PART I: *Blood Type and Aging: A Basic Primer*

ONE:
HOW THE BRAIN AGES   9

TWO:
BLOOD TYPE AND THE PATHS TO AGING   17

THREE:
FIGHTING AGING WITH NATUROPATHIC
AND BLOOD TYPE THERAPIES   28

PART II: *Individualized Blood Type Plans*

FOUR:
   BLOOD TYPE O   41

FIVE:
   BLOOD TYPE A   81

SIX:
   BLOOD TYPE B   124

SEVEN:
   BLOOD TYPE AB   167

Appendices

APPENDIX A:
   A SIMPLE DEFINITION OF TERMS   207

APPENDIX B:
   FAQs: THE BLOOD TYPE DIET   213

APPENDIX C:
   RESOURCES AND PRODUCTS   223

   INDEX   229

Aging

Fight It
with
the Blood
Type Diet*

INTRODUCTION

New Tools
to Fight
Aging

WHETHER YOU ARE YOUNG, OLD, OR SOMEWHERE IN between you want to stay strong, healthy, and mentally sharp for as long as possible. The Blood Type Diet can help you achieve that goal.

Aging: Fight It with the Blood Type Diet tailors the Blood Type Diet to the needs of those who are looking for ways to retain physical and mental vitality into their later years. If you think of the standard Blood Type Diet as the foundation, the guidelines in this book provide a more targeted overlay. Many medical conditions are a direct result of aging, either as a primary or a secondary factor. These dietary and lifestyle adaptations, individualized by blood type, supply additional ammunition to fight the aging process, by improving brain function, strengthening your immune system, and increasing metabolic and cellular fitness.

Here's what you'll find that's new:

- A disease-fighting category of blood type–specific food values, the **Super Beneficials**, emphasizing foods that have medicinal properties to strengthen immunity, reduce stress, and address specific medical conditions that are associated with aging.

- A more detailed breakdown of the **Neutral** category to limit foods that are known to have less nutritional value. Foods designated **Neutral: Allowed Infrequently** should be minimized or avoided.

- Detailed supplement protocols for each blood type that are calibrated to support you at every stage. They include protocols for **Basic Anti-Aging, Cognitive Improvement, Immune System Health,** and **Cellular Health**.

- A **4-Week Plan** for getting started that emphasizes what you can do right now to improve your condition and start feeling better immediately.

- Plus many strategies for success, checklists, and the answers to the questions most frequently asked about aging and the brain at my clinic.

The chemistry of blood type continues to provide important clues to the biological and genetic mechanisms that control health and disease. Medical doctors and naturopaths throughout the world are increasingly applying the blood type principles in their practices, with remarkable results.

I urge you to talk to your physician about the benefits of

incorporating individualized, blood type–specific diet, exercise, and lifestyle strategies into your current plan. I am confident that using the guidelines in this book will increase your fitness and vitality. Take the step now and use your blood type to your best advantage.

Why Blood
Type Matters

YOU ARE A BIOLOGICAL INDIVIDUAL.

Have you ever wondered why some people are constitutionally frail and susceptible to infection, while others seem naturally hardy? Why some people are able to lose weight on a particular diet, while others fail? Why some people age rapidly and show early signs of deterioration, while others are full of vitality into their later years?

We are all different. A single drop of your blood contains a biochemical signature as unique to you as your fingerprint. Many of the biochemical differences that make you an individual can be explained by your blood type.

Your blood type influences every facet of your physiology on a cellular level. It has everything to do with how you digest food, your ability to respond to stress, your mental state, the efficiency of your metabolic processes, and the strength of your immune system.

You can greatly improve your health, vitality, and emotional balance by knowing your blood type and by incorporating blood type–specific diet and lifestyle strategies into your health plan.

Be the biological individual you were meant to be!

PART I

Blood Type and Aging: A Basic Primer

O N E

How the
Brain Ages

I'VE NOTICED THAT AS PEOPLE REACH MIDLIFE, THEY often become resigned to a decline in mental clarity, as if it were a natural consequence of aging. They shrug off memory lapses, mid-afternoon fogginess, and the vague feeling that they're not as sharp as they used to be, believing that they can't expect to be as alert and focused at fifty as they were at twenty. The message of this book is that those assumptions about mental decline do not have to be true. You *can* change the way you age.

While aging inevitably takes a physical toll on all living creatures, a new scientific understanding of the brain and its pathways is demonstrating that most age-related decline in brain function can be prevented with long-term adherence to the proper diet, exercise, and lifestyle strategies. It's never too early—or too late—to start.

Why Do We Decline?

WHY DO SOME PEOPLE remain as sharp as a tack well into their senior years, while others begin to experience an unraveling of mental function as early as their forties and fifties? Until recently, most people thought the answer lay solely in genetics, and that little could be done to control the timing or rate of cognitive deterioration. But now it seems apparent that developmental and environmental factors are even more important.

In an intriguing study conducted by researchers at Children's Hospital in Boston and Harvard Medical School, the brain tissue of thirty individuals was examined to detect variations in genes involved in memory and learning, and in damage to those genes caused by the ordinary wear and tear of life. They found that damage patterns were strikingly similar for those between twenty-six and forty. They also found that after the age of seventy-three, almost all people showed more noticeable damage. But the big news was how wide the variations were in people between the ages of forty and seventy. The examiners concluded that lifestyle factors contributed to the rate of aging in the brain.

Scientists have isolated a number of factors that contribute to premature aging and brain deterioration. These include:

Mitochondrial Damage: Diseases of aging are increasingly being referred to as "mitochondrial disorders." About 95 percent of cellular energy production occurs in the mitochondria, the cells' energy powerhouses. Brain cells require a high level of energy metabolism to properly function. Damage to brain cell mitochondria, caused by free radical damage from toxins, infections, stress, and other wear and tear, can hasten aging.

Impaired Circulation: In assessing brain health, one factor stood out above all others: Across the board, whatever was good for the cardiovascular system was good for the brain. Keeping our systems well oxygenated is vital to continued brain health; heart disease, high blood pressure, and other circulatory problems clearly affect brain function. Impaired circulation resulting from atherosclerosis, heart disease, hypertension, and chronic inflammatory diseases causes injuries to cerebral blood vessels and brain cells. Mounting evidence suggests that the same factors involved in heart disease may also play a role in the development of Alzheimer's disease. Furthermore, recent research demonstrates that hypertension—high blood pressure—accelerates brain aging and predisposes the brain to strokes. Stroke is the third leading cause of death behind heart disease and cancer in our nation. More than 700,000 people suffer strokes each year; 200,000 of them suffer recurring strokes, causing further damage to their brains. Again, if the supporting metabolism is impaired, the brain suffers functional decline. The bottom line is, if the cardiovascular system is functioning well, there's a good chance the brain will be functioning well, too.

Hormonal Deficiency: As we age, the production of key hormones (DHEA, estrogen, testosterone) declines, contributing to poor energy metabolism in the brain.

Chronic Stress: Chronically high levels of cortisol, which destroy neurons and sap energy-producing ability by reducing effective glucose levels in the brain, are very detrimental to brain health. Chemical changes related to a decline in dopamine production slow metabolism in areas of the brain related to cognition. A key influence on dopamine decline is elevated levels of monoamine oxidase (MAO).

Nitric Oxide Impairment: Poor nitric oxide modulation impairs central nervous system function. Nitric oxide is a signaling molecule synthesized in neurons of the central nervous system, where it acts as a mediator with many physiological functions, including the formation of memory and the coordination between neuronal activity and blood flow.

Injury: Brain injury caused by accidents, or in sports such as soccer or boxing, contributes to early brain deterioration. A new series of studies show that former soccer players have declines in cognitive function in proportion to their use of their heads in propelling the ball. The aftereffects may not be apparent for months or even years, but the effects of injury can manifest at any time. These include headaches, impaired vision, dizziness, confused thinking, and altered personality. There are over five million Americans living with traumatic brain injury.

Tumor: Even a benign tumor can interfere with proper brain function.

Nutrient Deficiency: Key nutrient deficiencies—for example, a lack of essential fatty acids, folic acid, B_{12}, B_6, B_1—impair neuron stability and brain metabolism.

As you review this list, one thing should become clear: Each of the factors that contributes to premature brain decline can be mediated by diet, exercise, stress reduction, and healthful living. You have remarkable control when it comes to maximizing brain health at every stage of life.

The Alzheimer's Mystery

IS THIS HOPEFUL prognosis true of Alzheimer's disease? The ultimate thief of identity, Alzheimer's is a progressive form of dementia that has baffled scientists for the last century. As life expectancy has continued to increase, Alzheimer's disease has become more common: By some estimates, nearly 20 percent of people seventy-five to eighty-four suffer from this devastating condition. The shocking reality is that half of them have not seen their physicians or been clinically diagnosed and treated. Of those who have been diagnosed, a great number are not receiving any form of treatment.

Alzheimer's disease involves the parts of the brain that control thought, memory, and language. As the disease progresses, nerve fibers surrounding the memory center of the brain (the hippocampus) become tangled and are no longer able to carry messages to and from the brain. A second factor in Alzheimer's is the buildup of amyloid plaques—plaques that accumulate in the nerve cells and destroy them.

Scientists do not yet know what sets the deterioration in

motion, but a number of major studies are beginning to reveal lifestyle factors, such as diet, exercise, and stress reduction. Significant research has been done on the role of oxidative stress in damaging cellular molecules. Oxidative stress may play a role in the development of several neurodegenerative disorders. In the Alzheimer's diseased brain, in particular, such damage has been observed, especially in the late stages of the disease when both amyloid plaques and neurofibrillary tangles are present in abundance. Studies have shown that a reduction in free radicals through an antioxidant-rich diet improved cognition in older subjects.

Exercise is also emerging as a possible aid in preventing or delaying Alzheimer's. We know that regular exercise over a person's lifetime reduces the risk of developing high blood pressure, stroke, and cardiovascular disease, which in turn decreases the risk of Alzheimer's. However, new research suggests that exercise might actually shift the body's metabolic pathways toward the healthy processes that break down the amyloid precursor protein and prevent the buildup of amyloid deposits. The brain also benefits greatly from the increased blood circulation brought about and sustained by regular physical activity. Exercise is an excellent way to release stress and improve overall physical and emotional health.

Two studies are of particular interest. The first, conducted with 2,200 elderly Japanese American men in Hawaii, found that those who were sedentary or walked less than a quarter of a mile per day were nearly twice as likely to develop dementia and Alzheimer's disease compared to men who walked more than two miles per day. A second study of women seventy and older found that those who exercised regularly—including walking at an easy pace for at least 1.5

hours per week—appeared to have a lower risk of cognitive impairment than counterparts who were inactive. Women who engaged in the most activity—walking at least 6 hours per week—had a 20 percent decrease in risk of cognitive impairment compared to those who were inactive.

Several recent clinical studies have shown that dietary supplements can treat nutritional deficiencies in the elderly, boost their immune systems, combat short-term memory loss, reduce the risk of Alzheimer's, and improve overall health. The first, conducted at Memorial University of Newfoundland, concluded that supplementation with moderate amounts of eighteen vitamins, minerals, and trace elements improved short-term memory and overall cognitive abilities and strengthened immune system function in eighty-six elderly people treated over the course of one year. A separate study, published in *Neurology*, found that seniors with low levels of folate and vitamin B_{12} have an increased risk of developing Alzheimer's disease. A third study, published in *Nutrition*, showed that nutritional deficiencies greatly increase with age, and that supplement use helps eliminate these deficiencies in the elderly.

The evidence is mounting that supplementation with key nutrients can have a positive effect on the aging brain. However, a recent survey conducted by Harris Interactive found that people over sixty-five are least likely to discuss dietary supplements with doctors.

Message: Live Right to Protect Your Brain

THE BOTTOM LINE is that while aging baby boomers fear mental decline more than any other impairment, it is not by any means inevitable. We have the means to maintain the same mental clarity we had in youth well into our later years. Armed with the knowledge of what steps can be taken right now to prevent brain deterioration, we can fight the processes of aging.

Blood Type
and the Paths
to Aging

ANTIGENS PROTECT YOUR BODY AGAINST FOREIGN intruders such as bacteria, viruses, and parasites: When an antigen encounters a harmful foreign intruder, it creates antibodies against it. These antibodies serve as an early warning system. The next time the foreign intruder is encountered it will be attacked and destroyed.

Your blood type is also identified by its antigen. Blood type is expressed on every cell of your body and serves as a powerful guardian of your immune system. The antigen-antibody dynamic applies to all of the blood types—which is why transfusion with the wrong blood can be fatal. Blood Type O carries anti-A and anti-B antibodies and rejects anything with an A-like or B-like antigen. Type A carries anti-B antibodies, and Type B carries anti-A antibodies. Only Type AB carries no anti–blood type antibodies, which is why Type AB individuals can receive blood transfusions from anybody.

Many substances, such as bacteria, viruses, parasites, and some foods, actually resemble foreign blood type antigens, and it is the job of your blood type antibodies to recognize these intruders and target them for removal. If your blood type antigen fails to produce antibodies to foreign substances, the result is a weakened immune system. That's an important consideration for you at midlife, because as we age, the amount of protective antibodies produced by our antigens declines, thus weakening our immune defenses. This decline can be delayed by maintaining a healthy immune system.

Blood Type Antigens and Antibodies

BLOOD TYPE	ANTIGENS	ANTIBODIES
O	None— or "zero" (fucose)	You produce antibodies to Blood Types A, B, and AB. You can only receive Type O blood, but you can donate blood to all types. Because of this, Type O is often referred to as the universal donor. However, your system considers all things in nature that are A-like or B-like foreign.
A	A	You produce antibodies to Blood Type B. You can receive blood from Blood Types O and A, but you consider all things in nature that are B-like foreign.

BLOOD TYPE	ANTIGENS	ANTIBODIES
B	B	You produce antibodies to Blood Type A. You can receive blood from Blood Types O and B, but you consider all things in nature that are A-like foreign.
AB	A and B	Because both A and B antigens are present in your red blood cells, you don't carry antibodies for either. You can receive blood from Blood Types O, A, B, and AB. Because of this, Blood Type AB is often called the universal receiver.

Blood Type and Aging

YOUR IMMUNE SYSTEM has a life cycle, in which blood type plays a key role. Consider the life of the immune system as divided into three stages:

Stage 1: Education

As the immune system is first exposed to antigens, it begins to learn which are friends and which are foes. A functioning immune system will start to produce antibodies against the foes.

Stage 2: Maintenance

If the immune system has learned well, it will remain strong and healthy, effectively warding off foreign pathogens.

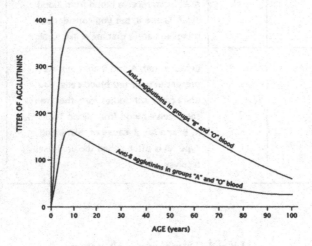

AGGLUTINATION AND THE PROCESS OF AGING

As we age, the amount of anti–blood type agglutinins in our blood diminishes, making us more susceptible to disease. A key factor in healthy aging is to maintain high levels of anti–blood type agglutinins.

Stage 3: Decline

As we age, our immune defenses weaken. Blood type antigens become less profuse and provide less protection against foreign antigens. The goal is to delay this final process. By encouraging a successful "education" stage, you can extend the "maintenance" stage of your immune system, and the final stage of decline will be delayed.

Are You a Secretor or a Non-Secretor?

ANOTHER FACTOR RELEVANT to your immune defenses is whether you are a secretor or a non-secretor. Although everyone carries a blood type antigen on their blood cells, about 80 percent of the population also secretes blood type antigens into body fluids, such as saliva, mucus, and sperm. These people are called secretors. The approximately 20 percent of the population that does not secrete blood type antigens into body fluids are called non-secretors. Being a secretor is independent of your ABO group; for example, there are both Type O secretors and Type O non-secretors.

Since blood type antigens are crucial to immune defense, being unable to secrete them into body fluids can place non-secretors at a disadvantage. In general, non-secretors are more vulnerable to immune diseases than secretors, especially when the disease is provoked by an infectious organism.

What Does Diet Have to Do with It?

SIMPLY PUT, THERE ARE chemical reactions between your blood type antigen and the foods you eat. That's because the proteins in foods have antigens as well, and these antigens are similar to the blood type antigens. If you eat food that contains or resembles a foreign antigen, your blood type antigen will create antibodies to it, and it will be rejected by your system.

Lectins are proteins in foods that are capable of binding

to antigens on blood cells, causing problems. The digestive impact of lectins is pervasive. They can interfere with the integrity of the digestive system, provoke inflammation, block digestive hormones, damage the intestinal lining, impair absorption, and interfere with protein digestion.

Many lectins are blood type–specific in that they show a clear preference for one kind of sugar over another and mechanically fit the antigen of one blood type or another. This blood type specificity results in their attaching to the antigen of a preferred blood type while leaving other blood type antigens completely undisturbed. At the cellular level, a common effect of lectins is to cause the sugars on the surface of one cell to cross-link with those of another, effectively causing the cells to stick together and agglutinate. Not all lectins cause agglutination. Many bacteria have lectinlike receptors that they use to attach to the cells of their host. Other lectins, called mitogens, cause a proliferation of certain cells of the immune system. But, in the most basic sense, lectins make things stick to other things.

Blood type–specific dietary lectins can wreak systemic havoc. They are directly correlated with three of the biggest age-related physiological problems—kidney failure, brain deterioration, and hormonal dysfunction. As we age, all of us experience a gradual drop in kidney function, defined as the volume of blood that is cleansed and recirculated into the bloodstream. This filtering system is very delicate—large enough for the various fluid elements of blood to move through, but small enough to prevent whole cells from passing. Lectins have been shown to stimulate the production of antibodies that are capable of destroying this delicate filter. Lectins that find their way into the bloodstream end up stimulating the production of antibodies, and the antibody/lectin complex can then lodge in the kidneys. The process is similar to having a clogged drain: As more and more agglutination occurs, less blood can be cleansed. Over time the filtration system ceases to function. Kidney failure is one of the leading causes of physical deterioration in the elderly.

Lectins play an equally destructive role in the brain. For example, the nerve cells of Alzheimer's patients exhibit a phenomenon called reactive plasticity—an aberrant sprouting of nonfunctional side connections between nerve cells. Much of this sprouting is characterized by the profuse production of glycosylated sugars, which are precisely the molecules lectins bind to. In fact, many dietary lectins have been used to map reactive plasticity pathways in brain samples from Alzheimer's patients.

The third way that lectins contribute to aging is their effect on hormonal functions. As people age, they have more trouble absorbing and metabolizing nutrients. Insulin resistance, which leads to type 2 diabetes, is a more common form of this trouble. Many lectins (most significantly the lectin found in wheat) act as false insulin, binding to the insulin receptors and blocking the action of true insulin, thus increasing resistance.

Most of my patients with chronic illnesses show the effects of some lectin activity. Knowing which lectins interact with your blood type and avoiding the foods that contain them can make a big difference to your overall health.

But it's not just a matter of avoiding harmful foods. Your blood type also recognizes foods that are beneficial—that support your unique chemical balance. The Blood Type Diet isn't only about saying no. It's also about saying yes!

Your Anti-Aging Blood Type Profile

KNOWING AND APPLYING the guidelines of the Blood Type Diet will help maximize your fitness as you age.

If You Are Blood Type O . . .

Overall, if you are following the Blood Type Diet and a regular exercise program, you are less vulnerable to the most common breakdowns that occur with aging. You have fewer risk factors for diabetes, heart disease, stroke, and cancer.

Your greatest vulnerabilities at this time of life involve inflammatory diseases, metabolic syndrome, and poor thyroid regulation—most of which can be mediated by diet.

Your optimal diet is a high-protein, low-fat diet with limited grains and lots of fruits and vegetables. Wheat should be avoided altogether.

You may have heard that a high-protein diet, such as the one recommended for Type O, can lead to excess calcium loss, which can be a concern as you age. However, this is not a danger for Blood Type O, since you have naturally high levels of intestinal alkaline phosphatase, an enzyme made by the intestine to split dietary fat and to help assimilate calcium. Furthermore, the high-protein Type O Diet actually causes an increase in intestinal alkaline phosphatase.

If You Are Blood Type A . . .

You are most vulnerable to a range of conditions triggered by depleted immune function and vulnerability to free radical damage, including cancer, cardiovascular disease, and strokes.

Your optimal diet is vegetarian with limited amounts of fish and fowl and greater amounts of healthy grains, beans, vegetables, and fruits. You should avoid red meat altogether and eat plenty of soy foods. Low levels of intestinal alkaline phosphatase and low hydrochloric acid make it difficult for you to digest meat and can make you vulnerable to osteoporosis. When you are not eating and living right for your type, you have a tendency to produce high levels of the stress hormone cortisol, which can place extra strain on your heart and contribute to brain decline.

If You Are Blood Type B . . .

You have a generally good prognosis for healthy aging, as long as you follow diet and exercise guidelines. Your optimal diet includes a balanced mix of meat, fish, dairy, fruits, and vegetables, with limited amounts of grains and beans. You should avoid chicken, corn, and wheat altogether, and you usually don't do well with soy foods.

Your greatest vulnerabilities at midlife are a tendency for slow-growing viral conditions, urinary tract infections, and insulin resistance—conditions usually mediated by diet. Like Type O, you have relatively high levels of intestinal alkaline phosphatase to aid protein digestion.

If You Are Blood Type AB . . .

You must negotiate your diet carefully, as you have aspects of both A and B blood. Like Type A, you have a higher risk for cancer, cardiovascular disease, and blood clots. Low levels of intestinal alkaline phosphatase affect your bone health. Type AB has the highest incidence of osteoporosis of all the blood types.

Your optimal diet involves utilizing the best of A and B. That means a healthy mix of fish, soy, some meat and dairy, fruits and vegetables, and specific grains. Like Type B, you should avoid chicken and corn.

Does Any One Blood Type Live Longer?

THERE HAVE NOT been many studies on the relative longevity of one blood type over another. However, three studies did show a slight increase in life span for Blood Type O over Blood Type A. Whether this is the result of a genetic link or simply the result of the fact that the modern high-fat diet and high-stress lifestyle is inherently more poisonous to Type A than Type O has not been determined. In any case, the studies are on small numbers of people and have not been replicated.

One older study looking at different rates of longevity between different nationalities saw the rate as being influenced by the percentage of Type A people in the population. Researchers stated that "innumerable influences of various types can cause diseases, primarily the high incidence of certain tumors in old age, climatic influences, overeating and malnutrition, and furthermore abuse of coffee, tea, tobacco, and alcohol, medicines, and insufficient movement. It can be assumed that wherever blood group A is prevailing, the genes of blood group A constitute a factor. The impact of the blood group genes varies as a function of the underlying disease, the effectiveness of the exogenic factors and the general constitution of the individual patient."

A third study of Italian dentists showed a higher incidence of Blood Type O among those who lived beyond seventy-five.

It has been my observation that Blood Type B also has a longevity advantage, as Type B individuals are, on average, a bit healthier than their counterparts. Since they tend to fall almost invariably between A and O with regard to disease susceptibilities, this tempering effect can be expected to translate into a higher percentage of Type B individuals attaining a more advanced age. This observation has been supported by at least one longevity study.

Remember, though, that these studies use populations that have done no interventions, such as diet or lifestyle modification. By following the Blood Type Diet, all blood types can better their odds of living longer, healthier lives.

THREE

Fight Aging with Naturopathic and Blood Type Therapies

YOUR BLOOD TYPE DIET IS DESIGNED TO WORK IN conjunction with medical and lifestyle strategies, including the use of supplements specifically tailored to blood type. I encourage you to share this information with your physician, making sure there are no conflicting effects with other medications that you may be taking.

There are four primary strategies for health and longevity of mind and body:

1. Four Keys to Fighting Aging with Blood Type Strategies

A healthy brain needs nutrition. That means eating right for your type and consuming sufficient amounts of key nutrients that promote brain health. Each of the Blood Type Diets includes plenty of antioxidant-rich foods that guard against free radical damage. The B vitamins are also crucial to nervous system function, especially folic acid, B_6, and B_{12}. Essential fatty acids found in fish oils provide fuel for brain metabolism and control inflammation involved in degenerative brain disorders.

Incorporating "brain foods" into a diet that is tailored for your specific needs creates a win-win scenario for healthy aging. The Blood Type Diet recognizes the variations in the ways individuals digest, metabolize, and utilize nutrients and efficiently eliminate wastes. These processes differ as people age, in conditions of chronic illness and as a result of genetically inherited biochemical differences—such as those related to blood type.

Many foods contain components that can react directly with the blood type antigens, resulting in inflammation and the production of toxins. Other foods address susceptibilities and strengthen our bodies against these weaknesses. When we consume these, we shift the odds in our favor.

Good digestion results not only from choosing the right foods for our bodies but also by keeping our digestive systems tuned and balanced so that the interplay of all important elements, such as digestive juices and hormones, is optimized for maximum nutrient absorption and regular elimination. As my father so aptly put it, "One man's food is another man's poison."

WILL SOY ROT YOUR BRAIN?

A flurry of concern about eating soy occurred in 2000 with the publication of a study by Dr. Lon White at the Pacific Health Research Institute in Honolulu. Dr. White charted the eating habits of 3,734 Hawaiian men over more than thirty years and made final assessments of their cognitive functioning (e.g., thinking, learning, memory), along with conducting tests for measuring brain atrophy, or shrinkage. His initial conclusion was that the men who ate two or more servings per week of tofu had steeper declines in brain function resulting in dementia. Could it be true that soy rots the brain?

Despite the dramatic results of his work, White recently told an interviewer, "I would be violating a cardinal rule if I said my data says you shouldn't eat tofu [or other soy foods]." While White believes his research is solid, the results, he says, "can't be turned into sweeping conclusions and the findings must be considered only preliminary." In addition, this same study concluded that the men who ate tofu had a 65 percent lower incidence of prostate cancer than their anti-soy counterparts.

Dr. White's study was of an observational nature in which the participants chose their lifestyles. He says his findings demand further investigation through more randomized trials. For example, study subjects (humans or animals) would be randomly divided; one group would be fed tofu and the other would not. The incidence of dementia in the two groups would then be measured and compared. A progression of such studies would either confirm or refute Dr. White's findings. He believes it will take at least ten years for a conclusion.

One could argue that if a causal effect existed between soy and Alzheimer's disease or increased brain aging, a greater incidence of Alzheimer's should exist in Japan and China, where tofu is eaten regularly—but no such effect has been documented. Another problem with White's findings is that they have not been duplicated in animal models. Though in general I am not fond of extrapolating conclusions from animals to humans, in this case it may be well worth noting that since White concluded that the soy isoflavone affected the synthesis of new DNA in the brain, its effects should be more marked in animals, who actually have more active brain DNA synthesis for a longer percentage of their life span than humans.

Finally, some researchers are questioning whether the link between tofu and brain aging may actually be another link between aluminum and brain atrophy. Although soy is low in aluminum, it does absorb quite a bit of it when cooked in aluminum cookware. The results of this preliminary investigation suggest that the aluminum concentration in soy products is increased slightly by cooking, particularly in an aluminum pot, and strongly (as much as fifteenfold) by some methods of tofu production.

> The bottom line: Soy should remain an important part of the diet, especially for Blood Type A, due to its demonstrable benefit in fighting cancer and cardiovascular disease. It may not be as helpful to the other blood types. Refer to your individual blood type section.

2. Exercise to Build Brain Power and Reduce Stress

The right kind of physical activity for your blood type can help you recover from stress and resist many of its harmful effects. As a rule of thumb, there is no substitute for proper physical exercise if you wish to experience optimal health. Studies clearly show that physical exercise significantly enhances the immune system's natural killer (NK) cell numbers and protective activities. This benefit occurs in males and females, and in people new to an exercise routine as well as to those who exercise regularly. Exercise also seems to be the great modulator against declines in NK activity with aging. In a few comparison studies of immune status between physically fit elderly individuals and young, not so physically fit sedentary controls, evidence suggests that habitual physical activity can enhance NK cell activity.

The question is, what is the best exercise? That depends on your blood type. Your goal should be to reduce the overall load on your system, not to exhaust it. If you exert yourself beyond your level of tolerance, exercise can actually act as a stressor. For example, overexercise will spike cortisol levels for Blood Type A individuals, furthering exhaustion.

On the other hand, Blood Type O thrives on vigorous aerobic exercise, while Blood Types B and AB fall somewhere in between.

Many factors interact to determine your tolerance for exercise, including proper nutrition, hydration, rest, prior training, level of fitness, and the stress in other parts of your life. An important factor influencing your level of tolerance is your blood type. All physical activity, even when it is not exhaustive, usually leads to elevated blood levels of stress hormones. However, following a period of training, most people will produce fewer stress hormones in response to exercise. In other words, once you get used to an exercise, it is not as stressful. That's what conditioning is all about.

3. Clean Out the Toxins

By balancing intestinal flora and improving digestive acid production, it is possible to restore gastrointestinal health and reduce the inflammatory responses of the system, giving it more strength to fight off the disease state. Friendly intestinal bacteria protect your cells, improve immune function, and have a positive effect on your ability to fully utilize the nutrients in the foods you eat. Blood type antigens orchestrate the proper balance of friendly bacteria in your system. Studies show that consumption of probiotics—lactic acid bacteria, or food cultured or fermented with these friendly microorganisms—does extend life and dramatically reduces a wide range of intestinal metabolites, such as indoles, polyamines, cresols, nitrates/nitrites, and carcinogens that we now know are counterproductive to good health. It is even more beneficial if you consume friendly bacteria specific to your blood type, since bacteria show favoritism for the sugars of one blood type over another.

4. Use Supplementation According to Your Blood Type

There has been a great deal of research on the effects of certain supplements to support overall health and brain function as we age. Among the most intriguing:

Mitochondrial Function and Repair

- *COQ-10:* Coenzyme Q-10 boosts mitochondrial cell function and reduces nerve cell death, increases the brain's cellular energy production, and reduces the damaging effects of free radicals. COQ-10 exerts a protective effect throughout the brain and may be useful in slowing a number of degenerative diseases.

- *Acetyl L-carnitine:* In conjunction with alpha-lipoic acid, acetyl L-carnitine reverses mitochondrial structural decay in the hippocampus region of the brain. It is needed to move fats into your mitochondria (the "energy" packet within the cell) where they can then be used as a source of energy. There is evidence that L-carnitine reduces insulin resistance. It lowers oxidative damage, improves mitochondrial function, and helps restore performance on memory-related tasks.

- *Alpha-Lipoic Acid:* Alpha-lipoic acid has tremendously positive benefits in conjunction with acetyl L-carnitine. At 100–600 mg per day, it can help improve sugar-handling capabilities. Lipoic acid is also a critical nutrient in energy metabolism and is an acclaimed and powerful antioxidant.

Healthy Brain Cell Activity

- *Methylcobalamin (active vitamin B_{12}):* This coenzyme form of vitamin B_{12} protects against age-related neurological disease.

- *Pantothenic acid (vitamin B_5):* Pantothenic acid helps activate neurotransmitters responsible for thought and memory.

- *Phospholipids:* Phospholipids help maintain the integrity of brain cell membranes.

- *Phosphatidylserine:* Found in trace amounts in lecithin, phosphatidylserine helps regulate the stress-induced activation of the HPA axis. In Europe, isolated as an extract, it has been approved as a drug to treat senility. It helps to maintain the integrity of the brain cell membrane by protecting it from breaking down, allowing essential nutrients to feed the brain cells. Although 100 mg per day is recommended for the healthy, up to 300 mg is suggested for those suffering from cognitive impairment or neurological disease.

- *Zinc:* Zinc aids brain metabolism. Zinc deficiency is common in people over the age of fifty.

- *Glutamine:* Glutamine aids alertness and clarity of thought, improves nerve health, and provides an energy source for the brain.

- *DHA (docosahexaenoic acid):* DHA is an omega-3 fatty acid, crucial to proper brain function.

Natural Antioxidants

- *Melatonin:* A naturally occurring hormone produced in the brain's pineal gland, melatonin declines with age, enhances cognitive function, and helps regulate the body's sleep cycle.

- *Vitamins A, C, and E:* These antioxidants protect against free radical damage and improve blood flow to the brain.

- *Green tea:* This potent antioxidant detoxifies the body and improves circulatory efficiency. It contains flavonoids and phenols that counteract free radical damage in the system.

- *Green "drink":* This typically includes a wide variety of sprouted seeds and grasses with high nutritional integrity and enzymatic activity. It may also contain antioxidant-rich foods.

Vascular Health

- *Ginkgo biloba:* Ginkgo improves blood flow to the brain, reduces strokes, enhances cognitive clarity, and may slow the progress of dementia. Ginkgo has been shown to help improve memory in healthy young people. It can aid the baseline condition of those with severe neurological deficit.

Nervous System Balance

- *Ginseng:* Ginseng boosts memory function, reduces the effects of stroke, and normalizes cortisol levels. It also increases energy and stamina. An abundance of research has demonstrated that it can enhance your response to physical or chemical stress, as well as have a beneficial effect on your central nervous, cardiovascular, and endocrine systems. Siberian ginseng (*eleutherococcus senticosus*) is suited to both males and females and has also been proven to help adapt your body to stressful circumstances.

- *NADH (nicotinamide adenine dinucleotide):* Through a series of reactions with acetyl and oxygen, NADH is able to produce energy. This energy is in the form of ATP, adenosine triphosphate. ATP is an energy-carrying molecule that exists in the cells of all living things. It serves as a kind of shuttle mechanism, delivering energy to living cells as they signal the need for it.

The Blood Type Diet plans in the next section contain protocols specifically calibrated to the needs of individuals of every blood type who want to fight premature aging.

ARE YOU READY TO START? Find your blood type section, and we'll get you on the right diet for your type.

PART II

Individualized Blood Type Plans

Blood Type

O

BLOOD TYPE O DIET OUTCOME: LIKE HAVING A NEW BRAIN

"I can hardly describe the change I have experienced on the Type O Diet. It is very near the top of the list of most important things that have happened to me in my life. I constantly have the thought, 'This is amazing, so this is how other people feel.' I wonder what I would have done in the last thirty years had I felt like this. As the months go by I continue to be amazed by the new territory in my psyche. I am grounded, clear, firm, and able, with lots of space to move around in and opportunity for choice. It's like having a new brain or an expanded being."

BLOOD TYPE O DIET OUTCOME: BETTER THAN EVER

"My chronic fatigue went away almost immediately on the Blood Type Diet. I have been able to give up 100 mg a day of Zoloft. I am sleeping a perfect 7.5 hours and then waking refreshed. My mind is clear and my memory is good. My aches and weakness are gone. My arthritis is gone. I have lost some weight without really watching my calories and feel sure that more will go as time passes."

Self-reported outcomes from the Blood Type Diet Web site (www.dadamo.com).

Blood Type O: The Foods

THE BLOOD TYPE O Fight Aging Diet is specifically adapted to provide the maximum nutritional support to fight many of the conditions associated with aging. A new category, **Super Beneficial**, highlights powerful disease-fighting foods for Blood Type O. The **Neutral** category has also been adjusted to de-emphasize foods that are less advantageous for you. Foods designated **Neutral: Allowed Infrequently** should be minimized or avoided entirely.

Your secretor status can influence your ability to fully digest and metabolize certain foods, so various adjustments in the values are made for non-secretors. If you do not know your secretor type, the odds are that you can safely use the "secretor" values, since the majority of the population (approximately 80 percent) are secretors. However, I urge you to get tested, since the variations are important for non-secretors who want to maximize the effectiveness of the Blood Type Diet.

Blood Type O

TOP 12 BRAIN POWER SUPER FOODS

1. lean, organic, grass-fed red meat
2. richly oiled cold-water fish (halibut, cod)
3. flax (linseed) oil
4. olive oil
5. walnuts
6. seaweeds
7. greens (spinach, collards, kale)
8. berries (blueberry, elderberry, cherry)
9. plums/dried plums
10. garlic
11. turmeric
12. green tea

The food charts are divided into three sections. The top of the chart suggests the average portion size and quantity per week or day, according to secretor status. These recommendations do *not* apply to the category **Neutral: Allowed Infrequently**; those foods should be eaten rarely, if at all. The charts also indicate differences in frequency for some foods, based on ethnic heritage. It has been my experience that this factor has an impact upon the individual's ability to fully digest certain foods. For the purposes of blood type food choices, persons of Hispanic heritage should follow the guidelines for Caucasians, and American Native peoples should follow the guidelines for Asians.

The middle section of the chart gives the food values. The bottom section lists variants based on secretor status.

For your convenience, we have included a number of product names (Ezekiel 4:9 bread, Worcestershire sauce, etc.). However, keep in mind that commercial formulations vary among brands and regions. For example, there are several forms of Ezekiel-bread, and not all may be right for your type. Even though a product may be listed as acceptable for you, always check its ingredients. Some products contain Avoid ingredients for your blood type. Of course, you may choose to make your own version of commercial products, such as bread and mayonnaise, using ingredients that suit your blood type. There are hundreds of delicious recipes for every blood type available on our Web site (www.dadamo.com) and in the book *Cook Right 4 Your Type: The Practical Kitchen Companion to* Eat Right 4 Your Type.

Meat/Poultry

Protein, in the form of lean, organic meat, is critical for Blood Type O and is the key to digestive health and immune function. Grass-fed beef, in particular, is high in omega-3 fatty acids and the essential fatty acid conjugated linoleic acid (CLA), which helps brain cell connectivity. Meat is also a good source of creatine, used in the manufacture of the energy compound adenosine. A high-protein diet also enables maximum metabolic fitness for Blood Type O, increasing lean muscle mass and improving basal metabolic rate. Choose only the best quality (preferably free-range) chemical-, antibiotic-, and pesticide-free low-fat meats and poultry.

BLOOD TYPE O: MEAT/POULTRY
Portion: 4–6 oz (men); 2–5 oz (women and children)

	African	Caucasian	Asian
Secretor	6–9	6–9	6–9
Non-Secretor	7–12	7–12	7–11
	Times per week		

SUPER BENEFICIAL	BENEFICIAL	NEUTRAL: Allowed Frequently	NEUTRAL: Allowed Infrequently	AVOID
Beef	Heart (calf)	Chicken		All commercially processed meats
Buffalo	Liver (calf)	Cornish hen		Bacon/ham/pork
Lamb	Mutton	Duck		Quail
	Sweetbreads	Goat		Turtle
	Veal	Goose		
	Venison	Grouse		
		Guinea hen		
		Horse		
		Ostrich		
		Partridge		
		Pheasant		
		Rabbit		
		Squab		
		Squirrel		
		Turkey		

Special Variants: *Non-Secretor:* BENEFICIAL: ostrich, partridge, pheasant, rabbit, squab; NEUTRAL (Allowed Frequently): lamb, liver (calf), quail, turtle.

Fish/Seafood

Fish and seafood represent a secondary source of high-quality protein for Blood Type O. There's a good reason fish is often called "brain food." In particular, richly oiled cold-water fish like cod, halibut, red snapper, and trout are SUPER BENEFICIAL for Blood Type O. These fish contain beneficial omega-3 fatty acids, such as docosahexaenoic acid (DHA) and eicosapentaenoic acid (EPA), which provide fuel for brain metabolism and help control inflammation. They are also good sources of creatine, which is used in the manufacture of the energy compound adenosine.

BLOOD TYPE O: FISH/SEAFOOD
Portion: 4–6 oz (men); 2–5 oz (women and children)

	African	Caucasian	Asian
Secretor	2–4	3–5	2–5
Non-Secretor	2–5	4–5	4–5
	Times per week		

SUPER BENEFICIAL	BENEFICIAL	NEUTRAL: Allowed Frequently	NEUTRAL: Allowed Infrequently	AVOID
Cod	Bass (all)	Anchovy	Eel	Abalone
Halibut	Perch (all)	Beluga	Flounder	Barracuda
Red	Pike	Bluefish	Gray sole	Catfish
snapper	Shad	Bullhead	Grouper	Conch

SUPER BENEFICIAL	BENEFICIAL	NEUTRAL: Allowed Frequently	NEUTRAL: Allowed Infrequently	AVOID
Trout (rainbow)	Sole (except gray) Sturgeon Swordfish Tilefish Yellowtail	Butterfish Carp Caviar (sturgeon) Chub Clam Crab Croaker Cusk Drum Haddock Hake Halfmoon fish Harvest fish Herring (fresh) Lobster Mackerel Mahimahi Monkfish Mullet Mussel Opaleye Orange roughy Oysters	Whitefish	Frog Herring (pickled/ smoked) Muskellunge Octopus Pollock Salmon (smoked) Salmon roe Squid (calamari)

SUPER BENEFICIAL	BENEFICIAL	NEUTRAL: Allowed Frequently	NEUTRAL: Allowed Infrequently	AVOID
		Parrot fish		
		Pickerel		
		Pompano		
		Porgy		
		Rosefish		
		Sailfish		
		Salmon		
		Sardine		
		Scallops		
		Scrod		
		Shark		
		Shrimp		
		Smelt		
		Snail (*Helix pomatia*/ escargot)		
		Sucker		
		Sunfish		
		Tilapia		
		Trout (brook/ sea)		
		Tuna		
		Weakfish		
		Whiting		

Special Variants: *Non-Secretor:* BENEFICIAL: hake, herring (fresh), mackerel, sardine; NEUTRAL (Allowed Frequently): bass, catfish, hailbut, red snapper, salmon roe; AVOID: anchovy, crab, mussel.

Dairy/Eggs

Most dairy foods should be avoided by Blood Type O. They are poorly digested and metabolized. Eggs can be eaten in moderation: They are a source of DHA and contain choline, which increases energy and enhances memory. Ghee (clarified butter) is one exception to the dairy rule because it's a good source of butyrate, which supports Blood Type O intestinal health. Do your best to find eggs and dairy products that are both hormone-free and organic. Try to find "high DHA" eggs.

BLOOD TYPE O: EGGS
Portion: 1 egg

	African	Caucasian	Asian
Secretor	1–4	3–6	3–4
Non-Secretor	2–5	3–6	3–4
		Times per week	

BLOOD TYPE O: MILK AND YOGURT
Portion: 4–6 oz (men); 2–5 oz (women and children)

	African	Caucasian	Asian
Secretor	0–1	0–3	0–2
Non-Secretor	0	0–2	0–3
		Times per week	

BLOOD TYPE O: CHEESE
Portion: 3 oz (men); 2 oz (women and children)

	African	Caucasian	Asian
Secretor	0–1	0–2	0–1
Non-Secretor	0	0–1	0
	Times per week		

SUPER BENEFICIAL	BENEFICIAL	NEUTRAL: Allowed Frequently	NEUTRAL: Allowed Infrequently	AVOID
	Ghee (clarified butter)	Egg (chicken/ duck)	Butter Farmer cheese Feta Goat cheese Mozzarella	American cheese Blue cheese Brie Buttermilk Camembert Casein Cheddar Colby Cottage cheese Cream cheese Edam Egg (goose/ quail)

SUPER BENEFICIAL	BENEFICIAL	NEUTRAL: Allowed Frequently	NEUTRAL: Allowed Infrequently	AVOID
				Emmenthal
				Gouda
				Gruyère
				Half-and-half
				Ice cream
				Jarlsberg
				Kefir
				Mile (cow/ goat)
				Monterey Jack
				Muenster
				Neufchâtel
				Paneer
				Parmesan
				Provolone
				Quark
				Ricotta
				Sherbet
				Sour cream
				String Cheese
				Swiss cheese
				Whey
				Yogurt

Special Variants: *Non-Secretor:* NEUTRAL (Allowed Frequently): egg (goose/quail); AVOID: farmer cheese, feta, goat cheese, mozzarella.

Oils

Olive oil, a monounsaturated oil, is SUPER BENEFICIAL for Blood Type O, and should be used as the primary cooking oil. Constituents in olive oil, such as flavonoids, squalenes, and polyphenols, act as powerful antioxidants. Flax (linseed) oil is high in alpha-linolenic acid, which has anti-inflammatory properties and aids brain cell connectivity. Be aware that some oils are high in omega-6 fatty acids, which can stimulate an inflammatory response. These include corn, cottonseed, peanut, and safflower oils. Secretors have a bit of an edge over non-secretors in digesting oils and probably benefit a bit more from their consumption.

BLOOD TYPE O: OILS
Portion: 1 tblsp

	African	Caucasian	Asian
Secretor	3–8	4–8	5–8
Non-Secretor	1–7	3–5	3–6
	Times per week		

SUPER BENEFICIAL	BENEFICIAL	NEUTRAL: Allowed Frequently	NEUTRAL: Allowed Infrequently	AVOID
Flax (linseed) Olive		Almond	Canola	Avocado Castor Coconut

SUPER BENEFICIAL	BENEFICIAL	NEUTRAL: Allowed Frequently	NEUTRAL: Allowed Infrequently	AVOID
		Black currant seed		Corn
				Cottonseed
		Borage seed		Evening primrose
		Cod liver		Peanut
		Sesame		Safflower
		Walnut		Soy
				Sunflower
				Wheat germ

Special Variants: *Non-Secretor:* BENEFICIAL: almond, walnut; NEUTRAL (Allowed Frequently): coconut, flax (linseed); AVOID: borage, canola, cod liver.

Nuts/Seeds

Overall, Blood Type O should limit intake of nuts and seeds in favor of high-quality animal protein. However, raw flax (seeds) is helpful for a strong immune system, providing beneficial omega-3 fatty acids. Walnuts are also SUPER BENEFICIAL. They are one of the best plant sources of omega-3 fatty acids.

BLOOD TYPE O: NUTS AND SEEDS
Portion: Whole (handful); Nut Butters (2 tblsp)

	African	Caucasian	Asian
Secretor	2–5	2–5	2–4
Non-Secretor	5–7	5–7	5–7
	Times per week		

SUPER BENEFICIAL	BENEFICIAL	NEUTRAL: Allowed Frequently	NEUTRAL: Allowed Infrequently	AVOID
Flax (linseed) Walnut (black/ English)	Pumpkin seed	Almond Almond butter Almond cheese Almond milk Butternut Filbert (hazelnut) Hickory Macadamia Pecan Pignolia (pine nut)	Safflower seed Sesame butter (tahini) Sesame seed	Beechnut Brazil nut Cashew Chestnut Lychee Peanut Peanut butter Pistachio Poppy seed Sunflower butter Sunflower seed

Special Variants: *Non-Secretor:* NEUTRAL (Allowed Frequently): flax (linseed); AVOID: almond cheese, almond milk, safflower seed.

Beans and Legumes

Essentially carnivores when it comes to protein requirements, Blood Type Os should minimize consumption of beans and legumes. Given the choice, get your protein from animal foods.

BLOOD TYPE O: BEANS AND LEGUMES
Portion: 1 cup (cooked)

	African	Caucasian	Asian
Secretor	1–3	1–3	2–4
Non-Secretor	0–2	0–3	2–4
		Times per week	

SUPER BENEFICIAL	BENEFICIAL	NEUTRAL: Allowed Frequently	NEUTRAL: Allowed Infrequently	AVOID
Fava (broad) bean	Adzuki bean Bean (green/ snap/ string) Black-eyed pea	Black bean Cannellini bean Garbanzo (chickpea) Jicama bean Lima bean Mung bean/ sprouts	Soy milk	Copper bean Kidney bean Lentil (all) Navy bean Pinto bean Tamarind bean

SUPER BENEFICIAL	BENEFICIAL	NEUTRAL: Allowed Frequently	NEUTRAL: Allowed Infrequently	AVOID
	Northern bean	Pea (green/ pod/ snow) Soy bean Soy cheese Soy, miso Soy, tempeh Soy, tofu White bean		

Special Variants: *Non-Secretor:* NEUTRAL (Allowed Frequently): adzuki bean, black-eyed pea, lentil (all), pinto bean; AVOID: fava (broad) bean, garbanzo (chickpea), soy (all).

Grains and Starches

Blood Type O does poorly with corn, wheat, sorghum, barley, and many of their by-products (sweeteners, etc.). In particular, the lectin in wheat produces gut inflammation and is a cause of celiac disease. Wheat is also a leading factor in Blood Type O's susceptibility to autoimmune thyroid disease, inflammation, and insulin resistance. Wheat sensitivity has been linked to neurological and behavioral problems. Non-secretors have even greater wheat sensitivity and should avoid oats as well.

The exceptions for Type O are sprouted seed breads, such as Essene (manna), usually found in the freezer section of your health-food store.

BLOOD TYPE O: GRAINS AND STARCHES

Portion: ½ cup dry (grains or pastas); 1 muffin; 2 slices of bread

	African	Caucasian	Asian
Secretor	1–6	1–6	1–6
Non-Secretor	0–3	0–3	0–3
	Times per week		

SUPER BENEFICIAL	BENEFICIAL	NEUTRAL: Allowed Frequently	NEUTRAL: Allowed Infrequently	AVOID
	Essene bread (manna)	Amaranth	Buckwheat	Barley
		Ezekiel 4:9	Millet	Cornmeal
		bread	Oat bran	Couscous
		Kamut	Oat flour	Grits
		Quinoa	Oatmeal	Popcorn
		Spelt	Rice (whole)	Sorghum
		(whole)	Rice (wild)	Wheat (re-
		Spelt flour/	Rice cake	fined/un-
		products	Rice flour	bleached)
		Tapioca	Rice milk	Wheat
		Teff	Rye (whole)	(semolina)
		100%	Rye flour/	Wheat (white
		sprouted	products	flour)
		grain	Soba noodles	Wheat
		products	(100%	(whole)
		(except	buckwheat)	Wheat bran
		Essene)	Soy flour/	Wheat germ
			products	

Special Variants: *Non-Secretor:* AVOID: buckwheat, oat (all), soba noodles (100% buckwheat), soy flour/products, spelt (whole), spelt flour/products, tapioca.

Vegetables

Vegetables provide a rich source of antioxidants and fiber, and the right selections can help Blood Type O balance immune functions. Fucose-containing seaweeds are SUPER BENEFICIAL in blocking lectin activity. They serve as a food source for healthy colon bacteria, thus reducing gut inflammation. Seaweeds also support thyroid function and are a good source of linolenic acid, which improves brain cell activity. Onions are high in quercetin, a flavonoid with potent antioxidant properties. Maitake mushrooms and green leafy vegetables promote healthy blood clotting and metabolic function. Antioxidant-rich vegetables, such as broccoli, spinach, and dark greens, protect against free radical damage.

An item's value also applies to its juice, unless otherwise noted.

BLOOD TYPE O: VEGETABLES Portion: 1 cup, prepared (cooked or raw)			
	African	**Caucasian**	**Asian**
Secretor Super/ Beneficials	Unlimited	Unlimited	Unlimited
Secretor Neutrals	2–5	2–5	2–5
Non-Secretor Super/Beneficials	Unlimited	Unlimited	Unlimited
Non-Secretor Neutrals	2–3	2–3	2–3
	Times per day		

SUPER BENEFICIAL	BENEFICIAL	NEUTRAL: Allowed Frequently	NEUTRAL: Allowed Infrequently	AVOID
Beets/ greens	Artichoke	Arugula	Brussels sprouts	Alfalfa sprouts
Broccoli	Beet	Asparagus	Cabbage	Aloe
Chicory	Dandelion	Asparagus pea	Olive (Greek/ green/ Spanish)	Cauliflower
Collards	Horse- radish	Bamboo shoot	Yam	Corn
Escarole	Kohlrabi	Beet		Cucumber
Kale	Lettuce (Romaine)	Bok choy		Leek
Mushroom (maitake)	Mushroom (abalone/ enoki/ oyster/ porto- bello/ straw/ tree ear)	Carrot		Mushroom (shiitake/ silver- dollar)
Onion (all)		Celeriac		Mustard greens
Potato (sweet)		Celery		Olive (black)
Seaweeds		Chili pepper		Potato
Spinach		Daikon radish		
Swiss chard	Okra	Eggplant		
	Parsnip	Endive		
	Pumpkin	Fennel		
	Turnip	Fiddlehead fern		
		Garlic		
		Lettuce (except Romaine)		
		Peppers (all)		
		Poi		
		Radicchio		

SUPER BENEFICIAL	BENEFICIAL	NEUTRAL: Allowed Frequently	NEUTRAL: Allowed Infrequently	AVOID
		Radish/ sprouts		
		Rappini (broccoli rabe)		
		Rutabaga		
		Scallion		
		Shallot		
		Squash		
		Tomato		
		Water chestnut		
		Watercress		
		Zucchini		

Special Variants: *Non-Secretor:* BENEFICIAL: carrot, fiddlehead fern, garlic; NEUTRAL (Allowed Frequently): lettuce (Romaine), mushroom (except shiitake), mustard greens, parsnip, potato (sweet), turnip; AVOID: Brussels sprouts, cabbage, eggplant, olive (all), poi.

Fruits and Fruit Juices

Blood Type O should eat lots of fruits rich in antioxidants, vitamins, and fiber. In particular, berries are super antioxidants and anti-aging catalysts. Blueberries have been studied for their anti-aging and antioxidant properties. Plums contain phytonutrients that reduce free radical damage. Bananas are excellent sources of potassium, promoting healthy circulation and lowering blood pressure.

An item's value also applies to its juices, unless otherwise noted.

BLOOD TYPE O: FRUITS AND FRUIT JUICES Portion: 1 cup			
	African	Caucasian	Asian
Secretor	2–4	3–5	3–5
Non-Secretor	1–3	1–3	1–3
	Times per day		

SUPER BENEFICIAL	BENEFICIAL	NEUTRAL: Allowed Frequently	NEUTRAL: Allowed Infrequently	AVOID
Blueberry	Banana	Boysenberry	Apple	Asian pear
Cherry	Fig (fresh/	Breadfruit	Apricot	Avocado
Elderberry	dried)	Canang	Currant	Bitter melon
(dark	Guava	melon	Date	Blackberry
blue/	Mango	Casaba	Grapes (all)	Cantaloupe
purple)	Pineapple	melon	Quince	Coconut
Plum		Christmas	Raisin	Honeydew
Prune		melon	Star fruit	Kiwi
		Cranberry	(caram-	Orange
		Crenshaw	bola)	Plantain
		melon	Strawberry	Tangerine
		Dewberry		
		Gooseberry		
		Grapefruit		
		Kumquat		
		Lemon		

SUPER BENEFICIAL	BENEFICIAL	NEUTRAL: Allowed Frequently	NEUTRAL: Allowed Infrequently	AVOID
		Lime		
		Loganberry		
		Mulberry		
		Muskmelon		
		Nectarine		
		Papaya		
		Peach		
		Pear		
		Persian melon		
		Persimmon		
		Pomegranate		
		Prickly pear		
		Raspberry		
		Sago palm		
		Spanish melon		
		Watermelon		
		Youngberry		

Special Variants: *Non-Secretor:* BENEFICIAL: avocado, pomegranate, prickly pear; NEUTRAL (Allowed Frequently): elderberry (dark blue/ purple); AVOID: apple, apricot, date, strawberry.

Spices/Condiments/Sweeteners

Many spices have medicinal properties. Turmeric activates an enzyme that prevents oxidation in the brain. Garlic is a super antioxidant that minimizes inflammation and helps prevent neurological disease. Cayenne pepper is anti-inflammatory. Ginger contains an antioxidant called zingerone, which appears to have brain protective properties. Many common food additives, such as guar gum and carrageenan, enhance the effects of lectins found in other foods and should be avoided. Use caution when using prepared condiments, as they often contain wheat.

SUPER BENEFICIAL	BENEFICIAL	NEUTRAL: Allowed Frequently	NEUTRAL: Allowed Infrequently	AVOID
Garlic	Carob	Agar	Apple	Aspartame
Parsley	Fenugreek	Allspice	pectin	Caper
Pepper	Ginger	Almond	Arrowroot	Carrageenan
(cayenne)	Horse-	extract	Barley malt	Cornstarch
Turmeric	radish	Anise	Chocolate	Corn syrup
	Parsley	Basil	Honey	Dextrose
		Bay leaf	Ketchup	Fructose
		Bergamot	Maple	Guarana
		Caraway	syrup	Gums
		Cardamom	Molasses	(acacia/
		Chervil	Molasses	Arabic/
		Chili	(black-	guar)
		powder	strap)	Juniper
		Chive	Rice syrup	Mace
		Cilantro	Senna	Maltodextrin
		(coriander	Soy sauce	MSG
		leaf)	Sucanat	Nutmeg
		Cinnamon	Sugar	Pepper
		Clove	(brown/	(black/
		Coriander	white)	white)

SUPER BENEFICIAL	BENEFICIAL	NEUTRAL: Allowed Frequently	NEUTRAL: Allowed Infrequently	AVOID
		Cream of tartar		Vinegar (except apple cider)
		Cumin		Worcester-shire sauce
		Dill		
		Gelatin, plain		
		Lecithin		
		Licorice root*		
		Marjoram		
		Mayonnaise		
		Mint (all)		
		Mustard (dry)		
		Oregano		
		Paprika		
		Pepper (peppercorn/red flakes)		
		Rosemary		
		Saffron		
		Sage		
		Savory		
		Sea salt		
		Stevia		
		Tamari (wheat-free)		
		Tamarind		
		Tarragon		

SUPER BENEFICIAL	BENEFICIAL	NEUTRAL: Allowed Frequently	NEUTRAL: Allowed Infrequently	AVOID
		Thyme		
		Vanilla		
		Vegetable glycerine		
		Vinegar (apple cider)		
		Wintergreen		
		Yeast (baker's/ brewer's)		

Special Variants: *Non-Secretor:* BENEFICIAL: basil, bay leaf, licorice root,* oregano, saffron, tarragon, yeast (brewer's); NEUTRAL (Allowed Frequently): carob, MSG, nutmeg, turmeric; AVOID: agar, barley malt, cinnamon, honey, maple syrup, mayonnaise, rice syrup, sage, soy sauce, stevia, sucanat, sugar (brown/white), tamari (wheat-free), vanilla, vinegar (apple cider).

* Do not use if you have high blood pressure.

Herbal Teas

Herbal teas can provide medicinal benefits and are excellent replacements for caffeinated drinks such as coffee, cola, and black tea. SUPER BENEFICIAL herbal teas for Blood Type O include ginseng, which can help improve cognitive function; sarsaparilla, which is anti-inflammatory; and dandelion, which aids liver function.

SUPER BENEFICIAL	BENEFICIAL	NEUTRAL: Allowed Frequently	NEUTRAL: Allowed Infrequently	AVOID
Dandelion	Chickweed	Catnip	Senna	Alfalfa
Ginseng	Fenugreek	Chamomile		Aloe
Sarsaparilla	Ginger	Dong quai		Burdock
	Hops	Elder		Coltsfoot
	Linden	Ginseng		Corn silk
	Mulberry	Hawthorn		Echinacea
	Peppermint	Horehound		Gentian
	Rosehip	Licorice		Goldenseal
	Slippery	Mullein		Red clover
	elm	Raspberry		Rhubarb
	Valerian	leaf		Shepherd's
		Skullcap		purse
		Spearmint		St. John's
		Vervain		wort
		White birch		Strawberry
		White oak		leaf
		bark		Yellow dock
		Yarrow		

Special Variants: None.

Miscellaneous Beverages

Green tea should be part of every Blood Type O's health plan. It is a potent antioxidant that improves intracellular energy production. Avoid or limit alcohol to an occasional glass of red wine. Try to eliminate coffee by slowly weaning yourself off and replacing it with green tea. The tea has less caffeine but more positive health benefits.

SUPER BENEFICIAL	BENEFICIAL	NEUTRAL: Allowed Frequently	NEUTRAL: Allowed Infrequently	AVOID

Tea (green)	Seltzer
	Soda (club)
		Wine (red)		Beer
				Coffee (reg/
				  decaf)
				Liquor
				Soda (cola/
				  diet/misc.)
				Tea, black
				  (reg/
				  decaf)
				Wine (white)

Special Variants: *Non-Secretor:* BENEFICIAL: Wine (red).

Supplements

THE BLOOD TYPE O DIET offers abundant quantities of important nutrients, such as protein and iron. However, properly calibrated supplements can provide important benefits. This may be especially true as we age. Recent clinical studies showed that dietary supplements can treat nutritional deficiencies in the elderly, boost their immune systems, combat short-term memory loss, reduce the risk of Alzheimer's, and improve seniors' overall health. The following supplement protocols are designed for Blood Type O individuals to improve brain health, cognitive function, and intracellular energy.

Note: If you are being treated for a medical condition, consult your doctor before taking any supplements.

Blood Type O: Basic Anti-Aging Protocol

Use this protocol for 4–8 weeks, then discontinue for 2 weeks and restart.		
SUPPLEMENT	ACTION	DOSAGE
High-potency vitamin-mineral complex (preferably blood type–specific)	Nutritional support	As directed
Alpha-lipoic acid	Protects against free radical damage; enhances insulin metabolism	50 mg, 1 capsule daily
Methylcobalamin (active vitamin B_{12})	Plays important role in homocysteine regulation, red blood cell production, and maintaining nerve integrity	500 mcg daily
DHA (docosahexaenoic acid)	Omega-3 fatty acid, which provides fuel for brain metabolism and helps control inflammation	100 mg, 1 capsule daily

SUPPLEMENT	ACTION	DOSAGE
Acetyl L-carnitine	A more bioavailable form of the amino acid L-carnitine, which is involved in many metabolic functions. As an antioxidant, protects neurons from damage caused by superoxide radicals	300 mg, 1 capsule daily

Blood Type O:
Cognitive Improvement Protocol

Use this protocol for 4–8 weeks, then discontinue for 2 weeks and restart.

SUPPLEMENT	ACTION	DOSAGE
Russian rhodiola (*Rhodiola rosea*)	Prevents stress-induced catecholamine activity	250 mg, 1–2 capsules, twice daily
Thiamine hydrochloride (vitamin B_1)	Supports nerve health	50 mg, 1 capsule, twice daily
Amla/Indian gooseberry (*Phyllanthus emblica*)	Antioxidant and anti-aging support	250 mg, 1–2 capsules daily
Folic acid	Improves cognitive function	400 mcg, 2 capsules daily

SUPPLEMENT	ACTION	DOSAGE
DMAE (dimethyl-amino-ethanol	May help to treat memory lapses, and even Alzheimer's disease, as well as certain movement disorders	100–300 mg, taken orally, twice daily

Blood Type O:
Immune System Health Protocol

Use this protocol for 4–8 weeks, then discontinue for 2 weeks and restart.

SUPPLEMENT	ACTION	DOSAGE
Larch arabinogalactan	Promotes digestive and intestinal health	1 tablespoon, twice daily, in juice or water
Caprylic acid	Has antifungal and antiseptic properties	350 mg, 1–2 capsules, twice daily away from food
Probiotic (preferably blood type–specific)	Promotes intestinal health	1–2 capsules, twice daily

Blood Type O: Cellular Health Protocol

Use this protocol for 4–8 weeks, then discontinue for 2 weeks and restart.		
SUPPLEMENT	ACTION	DOSAGE
Bladderwrack (*Fucus vesiculosus*)	Supports thyroid function; blocks the activity of complement; blocks lectins; prevents candida	100 mg, twice daily with meals
Coleus (*Coleus forskohlii*)	Enhances intracellular energy production through interaction with cellular second messengers	150 mg, 1 capsule, twice daily
Green tea	Improves cardiovascular and immune health; contains xanthines, which are important facilitators of intracellular energy production	1–3 cups daily

The Exercise Component

BLOOD TYPE O benefits tremendously from brisk exercise that taxes the cardiovascular and musculoskeletal systems. There is increasing evidence that vigorous exercise increases brain cells and guards against the negative effects of stress. Exercise increases brain-derived neurotrophic factor (BDNF), a protein critical to maintenance and repair of neural circuits.

Build a balanced routine of both aerobic and strength-training activities from the following chart. If you are not accustomed to exercising or you are suffering from a chronic condition, start slowly and do as much as you can, striving to increase your time and endurance as you gain flexibility and strength.

EXERCISE	DURATION	FREQUENCY
Aerobics	40–60 minutes	3–4 x week
Weight training	30–45 minutes	3–4 x week
Running	40–45 minutes	3–4 x week
Calisthenics	30–45 minutes	3 x week
Treadmill	30 minutes	3 x week
Kickboxing	30–45 minutes	3 x week
Cycling	30 minutes	3 x week
Contact sports	60 minutes	2–3 x week
In-line/roller skating	30 minutes	2–3 x week

3 Steps to Effective Exercise

1. Warm up with stretching and flexibility moves before you start your aerobic exercise.

2. To achieve maximum cardiovascular benefits, work toward an elevated heart rate that is about 70 percent

of your capacity. Once you reach the elevated rate, continue exercising to maintain that rate for twenty to thirty minutes. To calculate your maximum heart rate and performance level:

• Subtract your age from 220.
• Multiply the difference by .70 (or .60 if you are over age sixty). This is the high end of your performance.
• Multiply the remainder by .50. This is the low end of your performance.

3. Finish each aerobic session with at least a five-minute cooldown of stretching and relaxation moves.

Getting Started: The First Month

IF YOU ARE NEW to the Blood Type Diet, the following guidelines will introduce you to the Blood Type O regimen over a period of one month. Follow these recommendations as closely as possible, using a notebook to record your personal experiences with the diet. In addition to factors that are measurable in laboratory tests, take the time to note changes in your energy levels, sleep patterns, digestion, and overall well-being.

Blood Type O Brain-Boosting Diet Checklist

Eat small to moderate portions of high-quality, lean, organic, grass-fed meat several times a week for strength. ☐

Include regular portions of richly oiled cold-water fish. ☐

Consume little or no dairy foods.	☐
Eliminate wheat and wheat-based products from your diet.	☐
Limit your intake of beans principally to those that are BENEFICIAL.	☐
Eat lots of BENEFICIAL fruits and vegetables.	☐
Avoid stimulants found in caffeine (coffee, colas, etc.).	☐
Avoid coffee, but drink green tea every day.	☐

Week 1
Blood Type Diet and Supplements

- Eliminate your most harmful AVOID foods—wheat and dairy. These foods are the primary triggers for many health problems that afflict Blood Type O.
- Include your most important BENEFICIAL foods on a regular schedule throughout the week. For example, have lean red meat 5 times, and omega-3–rich fish 3 to 4 times, with lots of BENEFICIAL vegetables and fruit.
- Incorporate at least 1 SUPER BENEFICIAL food into your daily diet. For example, eat a snack of walnuts and cherries, or add seaweed to your salad.
- If you're a coffee drinker, begin to wean yourself by cutting your daily consumption in half. Substitute green tea instead.

Exercise Regimen

- Plan to exercise at least 4 days this week, for 45 minutes each day.
  2 days: aerobic activity
  2 days: weights

- If ill health is causing difficulty, start slowly and gradually increase your duration and intensity of activity. Exercise will energize you, not exhaust you. The important factor is consistency. Just do it—as much as you're able.
- Use your journal to detail the time, activity, distance, and amount of weight lifted. Note the number of repetitions for each exercise.

▪ WEEK 1 SUCCESS STRATEGY ▪
Exercise Your Mind

Is your brain like a muscle that can benefit from exercise? There is increasing evidence that new brain cells are generated in adults, giving rise to studies in neurobics, the study of mental exercise. A handy little workbook, *Keep Your Brain Alive*, by Lawrence C. Katz, Ph.D., and Manning Rubin (Workman Publishing, 1999), offers eighty-three simple little brain exercises to sharpen memory and create new cognitive pathways, using all five senses. The exercises include such activities as:

- Vary the order in which you accomplish daily tasks—for example, getting dressed after breakfast instead of before.
- Share a meal in silence, concentrating on the flavor and textures of the foods you eat.
- If you are normally in the driver's seat, hand the keys to your partner and sit in the back, experiencing the drive to work from another perspective.
- Shower with your eyes closed, negotiating only by touch.

- Brush your teeth with your nondominant hand.
- Learn Braille, utilizing the Braille codes in most public elevators and ATMs.
- Take an adventure or volunteer vacation to stretch your knowledge, imagination, and connection with the world.

Week 2

Blood Type Diet and Supplements

- Begin to eliminate the next level of AVOID foods—corn, potatoes, beans, and legumes.
- Eat at least 2 BENEFICIAL animal proteins every day, choosing from the meat, poultry, and seafood lists.
- Initially, it is best to avoid foods listed as NEUTRAL: Allowed Infrequently.
- Continue to incorporate SUPER BENEFICIAL foods into your daily diet.
- If you're a coffee drinker, continue to cut your coffee intake, substituting green tea.
- Manage your mealtimes to aid proper digestion. Avoid eating on the run. Make your meals relaxing, sit-down affairs. Eat slowly and chew thoroughly to encourage digestive secretions and better digestion.

Exercise Regimen

- Continue to exercise at least 4 days this week, for 45 minutes each day.
  2 days: aerobic activity
  2 days: weights
- If your work is sedentary, get in the habit of taking a couple of "movement" breaks during the day. Walk

around the block, or take the stairs instead of the elevator. If that is not possible, you can do light stretching exercises while seated.

■ WEEK 2 SUCCESS STRATEGY ■

Clean Up Your Internal Environment

Getting rid of toxins that inhibit metabolic activity and increase vulnerability to infections is crucial for Type O. The right blend of beneficial bacteria in the gut will help eliminate the interior atmosphere that encourages fungal growth. Start with a probiotic supplement, preferably blood type–specific. Your blood type antigens are prominent in your digestive tract, and, if you are a secretor, they are also prominent in the mucus that lines your digestive tract. Because of this, many of the bacteria in your digestive tract use your blood type as a preferred food supply. In fact, blood group specificity is common among intestinal bacteria with almost half of strains tested showing some blood type A, B, or O specificity. For more information about blood type–specific probiotics, go to the Web site www.dadamo.com.

Week 3

Blood Type Diet and Supplements

- When you plan your meals for week 3, choose BENEFICIAL or SUPER BENEFICIAL foods to replace NEUTRAL foods whenever possible. For example, choose lean, organic beef or buffalo over chicken, or blueberries over an apple.

- Eliminate all remaining AVOID foods.
- Liberally incorporate SUPER BENEFICIAL foods into your daily diet.
- Completely wean yourself from coffee, substituting green tea or herbal tea.

Exercise Regimen

- Continue to exercise at least 4 days this week, for 45 minutes each day.
  2 days: aerobic activity
  2 days: weights
- The most important thing is that you do what you can. If these recommendations are too vigorous, please adjust them to take any condition you may be experiencing into account.

• WEEK 3 SUCCESS STRATEGY •

Blood Type O Berry Brain Booster

Tufts University published a study involving several antioxidant-rich extracts such as spinach and blueberries. While all scored well in enhancing memory, only blueberries had a significant impact on improving motor skills like balance and coordination. While previous research has indicated that antioxidants may help lower the risk of cancer and heart disease, these new findings are the first to reveal a connection between potent antioxidants like blueberries and age-related declines. How do blueberries work? The authors of the Tufts study theorize that because blueberries keep the cell membranes healthy, they allow for more effective transport of important nutrients.

Blend together:
1 cup mixed berries (blueberries, blackberries,
elderberries)
1 cup light soy milk*
ice

---

*If desired, substitute Protein Blend 4 O, available through
www.dadamo.com.

Week 4

Blood Type Diet and Supplements

- Continue at the week 3 level, focusing on BENEFICIAL and SUPER BENEFICIAL foods.
- Evaluate the first 4 weeks and make adjustments.

Exercise Regimen

- Continue at the week 3 level.
- Review your progress, noting in your journal improvements in strength, flexibility, and overall energy. Determine which exercise regimen has worked for you, including time of day, setting, and activity level.

■ WEEK 4 SUCCESS STRATEGY ■
Tips for Type O Seniors

Mobility is a primary issue for seniors, and this is especially true for Blood Type Os, who thrive on physical activity. Pay careful attention to the following strategies:

- Maintain a high-protein diet, using protein shakes as supplements, if you need to. Protein is the key for preventing arthritis and inflammatory conditions, which are problems for Blood Type O. It is also the key for maintaining healthy bones and muscle mass.
- If you have painful rheumatoid arthritis or inflammation, avoid using nonsteroidal anti-inflammatory drugs, such as ibuprofen and naprosin. These are known to cause peptic ulcers in Blood Type O patients.
- Think twice about undergoing elective surgery that might keep you off your feet for a few days. Studies show that for the average elderly person, one week of hospitalization is equivalent to one year of lost activity.
- Avoid denture stomatitis, an inflammation of the mouth that occurs in denture wearers, which has been found to be most prevalent and severe in Blood Type O. One of the more common causes of dental stomatitis is infection with the parasite Candida albicans. Prevent candida by following the Blood Type O Diet and anti-inflammatory supplement protocol.

FIVE

Blood Type

BLOOD TYPE A DIET OUTCOME: AWAKENING

"I have tried a lot of lifestyle changes in the past, and this one really works. I used to get tired by four in the afternoon. It was hard for me to get home because I would fall asleep behind the wheel. My job demanded a lot of energy and by the afternoon I was gone. On the Type A diet, thinking and short-term memory have returned."

BLOOD TYPE A DIET OUTCOME: THE OLD FEELING'S BACK

"I am a forty-six-year-old teacher, and I'd reached the end of my endurance. I was tired and stressed and feeling lousy. I was asking questions of myself, like 'What's wrong with you? You aren't that old to feel like you are eighty-seven.' My girlfriend turned me on to your book, and everything fell into place with the Type A Diet. Thank you! I always knew that there was more to blood type than met the eye."

Self-reported outcomes from the Blood Type Diet Web site (www.dadamo.com).

Blood Type A: The Foods

THE BLOOD TYPE A Fight Aging Diet is specifically adapted to provide the maximum nutritional support to fight many of the conditions associated with aging. A new category, **Super Beneficial**, highlights powerful disease-fighting foods for Blood Type A. The **Neutral** category has also been adjusted to de-emphasize foods that are less advantageous for you. Foods designated **Neutral: Allowed Infrequently** should be minimized or avoided entirely.

Your secretor status can influence your ability to fully digest and metabolize certain foods, so various adjustments in the values are made for non-secretors. If you do not know your secretor type, the odds are that you can safely use the "secretor" values, since the majority of the population (approximately 80 percent) are secretors. However, I urge you to get tested, since the variations are important for non-secretors who want to maximize the effectiveness of the Blood Type Diet.

The food charts are divided into three sections. The top of the chart suggests the average portion size and quantity per week or day, according to secretor status. These recommendations do *not* apply to the category **Neutral: Allowed Infrequently**; those foods should be eaten rarely, if at all. The charts also indicate differences in frequency for some foods, based on ethnic heritage. It has been my experience that this factor has an impact upon the individual's ability to fully digest certain foods. For the purposes of blood type food choices, persons of Hispanic heritage should follow the guidelines for Caucasians, and American Native peoples should follow the guidelines for Asians.

Blood Type A

TOP 12 BRAIN POWER SUPER FOODS

1. walnuts
2. richly oiled cold-water fish (salmon, sardines)
3. berries (blueberry, cherry, elderberry)
4. flax (linseed) oil
5. onion
6. dark leafy greens (spinach, kale, Swiss chard)
7. soy-based foods
8. olive oil
9. ginger
10. garlic
11. turmeric
12. green tea

The middle section of the chart gives the food values. The bottom section lists variants based on secretor status.

For your convenience, we have included a number of product names (Ezekiel 4:9 bread, Worcestershire sauce, etc.). However, keep in mind that commercial formulations vary among brands and regions. For example, there are several forms of Ezekiel 4:9 bread, and not all may be right for your type. Even though a product may be listed as acceptable for you, always check its ingredients. Some products contain **Avoid** ingredients for your blood type. Of course, you may choose to make your own version of commercial products, such as bread and mayonnaise, using ingredients that suit your blood type. There are hundreds of delicious recipes for every blood type available on our Web site (www.dadamo.com) and in the book *Cook Right 4 Your Type: The Practical Kitchen Companion to* Eat Right 4 Your Type.

Meat/Poultry

Blood Type A lacks some of the enzymes and stomach acids needed to effectively digest animal protein. When you overconsume meat, the undigested by-products can foster a toxic intestinal environment. For this reason, Blood Type As should derive most of their protein from nonmeat sources. Non-secretors have a small advantage over secretors in the ability to digest animal protein but should still derive most of their protein from foods other than meat. Choose only the best quality (preferably free-range), chemical-, antibiotic-, and pesticide-free low-fat meats and poultry.

BLOOD TYPE A: MEAT/POULTRY Portion: 4–6 oz (men); 2–5 oz (women and children)			
	African	**Caucasian**	**Asian**
Secretor	0–2	0–3	0–3
Non-Secretor	2–5	2–4	2–3
		Times per week	

SUPER BENEFICIAL	BENEFICIAL	NEUTRAL: Allowed Frequently	NEUTRAL: Allowed Infrequently	AVOID
		Chicken		All commercially processed meats
		Cornish hen		Bacon/ham/pork
		Grouse		Beef
		Guinea hen		Buffalo
		Ostrich		Duck
		Squab		Goat
		Turkey		Goose
				Heart (beef)
				Horse
				Lamb
				Liver (calf)
				Mutton
				Partridge
				Pheasant
				Quail
				Rabbit
				Squirrel
				Sweetbreads
				Turtle
				Veal
				Venison

Special Variants: *Non-Secretor:* BENEFICIAL: turkey; NEUTRAL (Allowed Frequently): duck, goat, goose, lamb, mutton, partridge, pheasant, quail, rabbit, turtle.

Fish/Seafood

Fish and seafood represent a nutritious source of protein for Blood Type A. SUPER BENEFICIAL are the richly oiled cold-water fish, such as cod, mackerel, salmon, sardines, and trout. These are high in omega-3 fatty acids, such as docosahexaenoic acid (DHA) and eicosapentaenoic acid (EPA), which provide fuel for brain metabolism. There's a reason why fish is sometimes called "brain food."

BLOOD TYPE O: FISH/SEAFOOD
Portion: 4–6 oz (men); 2–5 oz (women and children)

	African	Caucasian	Asian
Secretor	1–3	1–3	1–3
Non-Secretor	2–5	2–5	2–4
	Times per week		

SUPER BENEFICIAL	BENEFICIAL	NEUTRAL: Allowed Frequently	NEUTRAL: Allowed Infrequently	AVOID
Cod	Carp	Abalone		Anchovy
Mackerel	Monkfish	Bass (sea)		Barracuda
Salmon	Perch	Bullhead		Bass
Sardine	(silver/	Butterfish		(bluegill/
Trout	yellow)	Chub		striped)
(rainbow)	Pickerel	Croaker		Beluga

SUPER BENEFICIAL	BENEFICIAL	NEUTRAL: Allowed Frequently	NEUTRAL: Allowed Infrequently	AVOID
	Pollock	Cusk		Bluefish
	Red	Drum		Catfish
	snapper	Halfmoon		Caviar
	Snail (*Helix*	fish		(sturgeon)
	pomatia/	Mahimahi		Clam
	escargot)	Mullet		Conch
	Trout (sea)	Muskellunge		Crab
	Whitefish	Orange		Crayfish
	Whiting	roughy		Eel
		Parrot fish		Flounder
		Perch (white)		Frog
		Pike		Gray sole
		Pompano		Grouper
		Porgy		Haddock
		Rosefish		Hake
		Sailfish		Halibut
		Salmon roe		Harvest fish
		Scrod		Herring
		Shark		(fresh/
		Smelt		pickled/
		Sturgeon		smoked)
		Sucker		Lobster
		Sunfish		Mussel
		Swordfish		Octopus
		Tilapia		Opaleye
		Trout (brook)		Oysters
		Tuna		

SUPER BENEFICIAL	BENEFICIAL	NEUTRAL: Allowed Frequently	NEUTRAL: Allowed Infrequently	AVOID
		Weakfish Yellowtail		Salmon (smoked) Scallops Scup Shad Shrimp Sole Squid (calamari) Tilefish

Special Variants: *Non-Secretor:* BENEFICIAL: chub, cusk, drum, half-moon fish, harvest fish, mullet, muskellunge, perch (white), pompano, rosefish, sailfish, sucker, swordfish, trout (brook); NEUTRAL (Allowed Frequently): anchovy, bass (bluegill), beluga, bluefish, caviar (sturgeon), flounder, frog, gray sole, grouper, haddock, hake, halibut, herring (fresh), mussel, octopus, opaleye, scallops, scup, shad, tilefish.

Dairy/Eggs

Dairy foods should mostly be avoided by Blood Type A, with the exception of a moderate intake of cultured dairy (kefir, yogurt), which can enhance immunity. Yogurt is a good source of pantothenic acid, a B vitamin essential for energy metabolism and cognitive function. Eggs can be eaten in moderation. They are a source of DHA and contain choline, which increases energy and enhances memory. Do your best to find eggs and dairy products that are both hormone-free and organic.

BLOOD TYPE A: EGGS

Portion: 1 egg

	African	Caucasian	Asian
Secretor	1–3	1–3	1–3
Non-Secretor	2–3	2–5	2–4
		Times per week	

BLOOD TYPE A: MILK AND YOGURT

Portion: 4–6 oz (men); 2–5 oz (women and children)

	African	Caucasian	Asian
Secretor	0–1	1–3	0–3
Non-Secretor	0–1	1–2	0–2
		Times per week	

BLOOD TYPE A: CHEESE

Portion: 3 oz (men); 2 oz (women and children)

	African	Caucasian	Asian
Secretor	0–2	1–3	0–2
Non-Secretor	0	0–1	0–1
		Times per week	

SUPER BENEFICIAL	BENEFICIAL	NEUTRAL: Allowed Frequently	NEUTRAL: Allowed Infrequently	AVOID
		Egg (chicken/ duck/ goose/ quail)	Feta	American cheese
		Farmer cheese	Goat cheese	Blue cheese
		Ghee (clarified butter)	Milk (goat)	Brie
		Kefir	Sour cream	Butter
		Mozzarella		Buttermilk
		Paneer		Camembert
		Ricotta		Casein
		Yogurt		Cheddar
				Colby
				Cottage cheese
				Cream cheese
				Edam
				Emmenthal
				Gouda
				Gruyère
				Half-and-half
				Ice cream
				Jarlsberg
				Milk (cow)
				Monterey Jack
				Muenster
				Neufchâtel

SUPER BENEFICIAL	BENEFICIAL	NEUTRAL: Allowed Frequently	NEUTRAL: Allowed Infrequently	AVOID
				Parmesan Provolone Sherbet Swiss cheese Whey

Special Variants: *Non-Secretor:* NEUTRAL (Allowed Frequently): cottage cheese, whey; AVOID: milk (goat), sour cream.

Oils

Olive oil, a monounsaturated fat, is SUPER BENEFICIAL for Blood Type A and should be used as a primary cooking oil. Constituents in olive oil, such as flavonoids, squalenes, and polyphenols, act as powerful antioxidants. Flax (linseed) oil is high in alpha-linolenic acid, which aids brain cell connectivity. Walnut oil has been shown to lower triglycerides and may help to reduce the risk of coronary heart disease.

BLOOD TYPE A: OILS
Portion: 1 tblsp

	African	Caucasian	Asian
Secretor	5–8	5–8	5–8
Non-Secretor	3–7	3–7	3–6
	Times per week		

SUPER BENEFICIAL	BENEFICIAL	NEUTRAL: Allowed Frequently	NEUTRAL: Allowed Infrequently	AVOID
Flax (linseed) Olive Walnut	Black currant seed	Almond Avocado Borage seed Cod liver Evening primrose Safflower Sesame Soy Sunflower Wheat germ	Canola	Castor Coconut Corn Cottonseed Peanut

Special Variants: *Non-Secretor:* BENEFICIAL: cod liver, sesame; NEUTRAL (Allowed Frequently): peanut; AVOID: safflower.

Nuts/Seeds

Nuts and seeds can serve as an important secondary source of protein for Blood Type A. Laboratory research has identified at least five natural phytochemicals in nuts that regulate the immune system and act as antioxidants. SUPER BENEFICIAL for Blood Type A are raw flaxseeds and walnuts, which are high in omega-3 fatty acids.

BLOOD TYPE A: NUTS/SEEDS

Portion: Whole (handful); Nut Butters (2 tblsp)

	African	Caucasian	Asian
Secretor	4–7	4–7	4–7
Non-Secretor	5–7	5–7	5–7
	Times per week		

SUPER BENEFICIAL	BENEFICIAL	NEUTRAL: Allowed Frequently	NEUTRAL: Allowed Infrequently	AVOID
Flax (linseed) Walnut (black/ English)	Peanut Peanut butter Pumpkin seed	Almond Almond butter Almond cheese Almond milk Beechnut Butternut Chestnut Filbert (hazelnut) Hickory nut Lychee Macadamia nut Pecan Pignolia (pine nut) Poppy seed	Safflower seed Sesame butter (tahini) Sesame seed	Brazil nut Cashew Pistachio

SUPER BENEFICIAL	BENEFICIAL	NEUTRAL: Allowed Frequently	NEUTRAL: Allowed Infrequently	AVOID
		Sunflower butter Sunflower seed		

Special Variants: *Non-Secretor:* AVOID: safflower seed, sunflower butter, sunflower seed.

Beans and Legumes

Blood Type A thrives on vegetable proteins found in many beans and legumes, although a few beans contain immunoreactive proteins and should be avoided. SUPER BENEFICIAL beans and legumes for Blood Type A include soy beans and their by-products. They are a good source of essential amino acids and contain isoflavones that can inhibit inflammation-inducing selectins from being overexpressed on the blood vessels. Soy also contains phospholipids, which help maintain brain cell membranes.

BLOOD TYPE A: BEANS AND LEGUMES
Portion: 1 cup (cooked)

	African	Caucasian	Asian
Secretor	5–7	5–7	5–7
Non-Secretor	3–5	3–5	3–5
	Times per week		

SUPER BENEFICIAL	BENEFICIAL	NEUTRAL: Allowed Frequently	NEUTRAL: Allowed Infrequently	AVOID
Soy bean	Adzuki	Cannellini		Copper
Soy, miso	bean	bean		bean
Soy, tempeh	Bean	Jicama bean		Garbanzo
	(green/	Mung bean/		(chickpea)
	snap/	sprouts		Kidney bean
	string)	Northern		Lima bean
	Black bean	bean		Navy bean
	Black-eyed	Pea (green/		Tamarind
	pea	pod/snow)		bean
	Fava	White bean		
	(broad)			
	bean			
	Lentil (all)			
	Pinto bean			
	Soy cheese			
	Soy milk			
	Soy, tofu			

Special Variants: *Non-Secretor:* NEUTRAL (Allowed Frequently): adzuki bean, bean (green/snap/string), black bean, black-eyed pea, copper bean, fava (broad) bean, kidney bean, navy bean, soy bean and products.

Grains and Starches

Blood Type A benefits from a moderate consumption of grains. However, those who suffer from frequent colds and infections, or who have a serious illness, should limit or avoid wheat and corn. This is especially important for non-secretors.

BLOOD TYPE A: GRAINS AND STARCHES

Portion: ½ cup dry (grains or pastas); 1 muffin; 2 slices of bread

	African	Caucasian	Asian
Secretor	7–10	7–9	7–10
Non-Secretor	5–7	5–7	5–7
		Times per week	

SUPER BENEFICIAL	BENEFICIAL	NEUTRAL: Allowed Frequently	NEUTRAL: Allowed Infrequently	AVOID
	Amaranth	Barley	Cornmeal	Teff
	Buckwheat	Kamut	Couscous	Wheat bran
	Essene	Quinoa	Grits	Wheat germ
	bread	Rice (wild)	Millet	
	(manna)	Rice cake	Popcorn	
	Ezekiel 4:9	Rice flour/	Tapioca	
	bread	products	Wheat	
	Oat bran	Rice milk	(whole)	
	Oat flour	Rye flour/		
	Oatmeal	products		
	Rice	Sorghum		
	(whole)	Spelt (whole)		
	Rice bran	Spelt flour/		
	Rye (whole)	products		
	Soy flour/	Wheat (re-		
	products	fined-un-		
		bleached)		
		Wheat		
		(semolina)		

SUPER BENEFICIAL	BENEFICIAL	NEUTRAL: Allowed Frequently	NEUTRAL: Allowed Infrequently	AVOID
	Soba noodles (100% buckwheat)	Wheat (white flour) 100% sprouted grain products (except Essene, Ezekiel)		

Special Variants: *Non-Secretor:* NEUTRAL (Allowed Frequently): buckwheat, Ezekiel 4:9 bread, oat (all), soba noodles (100% buckwheat), soy flour/products, teff; AVOID: cornmeal, couscous, grits, popcorn, wheat (all).

Vegetables

Vegetables can be a first line of defense against chronic illness, providing a rich source of nutrients, including antioxidants and fiber. Blood Type A SUPER BENEFICIALS include onions, which are high in quercetin and other antioxidants that decrease oxidative stress and increase glutathione, which protects cells. Broccoli contains allyl methyl trisulfide and dithiolthiones, which increase the activity of enzymes involved in detoxification of carcinogens. Spinach, kale, Swiss chard, and escarole contain excellent antioxidants. Okra and parsnips are very good sources of vitamin C and folic acid. Dandelions are renowned for their vitamin- and mineral-packed qualities, helpful to cardiovascular and neurological function. SUPER BENEFICIAL vegetables also help detoxify xenobiotic compounds in the liver.

Tomatoes contain a lectin that reacts with the saliva and digestive juices of Blood Type A secretors, although it does not appear to react with non-secretors. Yams are typically high in the amino acid phenylalanine, which inactivates intestinal alkaline phosphatase (already quite low in Blood Type A) and should be minimized or avoided completely.

An item's value also applies to its juices, unless otherwise noted.

BLOOD TYPE A: VEGETABLES Portion: 1 cup, prepared (cooked or raw)			
	African	**Caucasian**	**Asian**
Secretor Super/ Beneficials	Unlimited	Unlimited	Unlimited
Secretor Neutrals	2–5	2–5	2–5
Non-Secretor Super/Beneficials	Unlimited	Unlimited	Unlimited
Non-Secretor Neutrals	2–5	2–5	2–5
		Times per day	

SUPER BENEFICIAL	BENEFICIAL	NEUTRAL: Allowed Frequently	NEUTRAL: Allowed Infrequently	AVOID
Broccoli	Alfalfa	Arugula	Corn	Cabbage
Dandelion	sprouts	Asparagus	Olive	Eggplant
Escarole	Aloe	Asparagus	(green)	Mushroom
Kale	Artichoke	pea	Pickle	(shiitake)
Okra	Beet	Bamboo	(in brine)	Olive (black/
Onion (all)	Beet greens	shoot	Squash (all)	Greek/
Parsnip	Carrot	Beet		Spanish)
Spinach	Chicory	Bok choy		Peppers (all)
Swiss chard	Celery	Brussels		Pickle (in
	Collards	sprouts		vinegar)
	Garlic	Cabbage		Potato
	Horse-	(juice)*		Potato
	radish	Cauliflower		(sweet)
	Kohlrabi	Celeriac		Rhubarb
	Leek	Cucumber		Tomato
	Lettuce	Daikon		Yam
	(Romaine)	radish		Yucca
	Mushroom	Endive		
	(maitake/	Fennel		
	silver	Fiddlehead		
	dollar)	fern		
	Pumpkin	Lettuce		
	Rappini	(except		
	(broccoli	Romaine)		
	rabe)	Mung bean/		
		sprouts		

SUPER BENEFICIAL	BENEFICIAL	NEUTRAL: Allowed Frequently	NEUTRAL: Allowed Infrequently	AVOID
	Turnip	Mushroom (abalone/ enoki/ oyster/ portobello/ straw/tree ear) Mustard greens Oyster plant Poi Radicchio Radish/ sprouts Rutabaga Scallion Seaweed Shallot Taro Water chestnut Watercress Zucchini		

Special Variants: *Non-Secretor:* NEUTRAL (Allowed Frequently): alfalfa sprouts, aloe, carrot, celery, eggplant, garlic, horseradish, lettuce (Romaine), mushroom (maitake/shiitake), peppers (all), potato (sweet), rappini, tomato; AVOID: cabbage (juice), mushroom (silver dollar), pickle (in brine).

* To obtain the benefits of cabbage juice, it must be consumed within one minute of juicing.

Fruits and Fruit Juices

Fruits are rich in antioxidants, especially blueberries, elderberries, cherries, and blackberries. Blueberries have been studied for their anti-aging and antioxidant properties. Plums and prunes are high in the phytonutrients neochlorogenic and chlorogenic acids. These substances are classified as phenols, and their function as antioxidants has been well-documented. Several fruits, such as bananas and oranges, contain Blood Type A–reactive lectins and should be avoided.

An item's value also applies to its juice, unless otherwise noted.

BLOOD TYPE A: FRUITS AND FRUIT JUICES
Portion: 1 cup

	African	Caucasian	Asian
Secretor	2–4	3–4	3–4
Non-Secretor	2–3	2–3	2–3
		Times per day	

SUPER BENEFICIAL	BENEFICIAL	NEUTRAL: Allowed Frequently	NEUTRAL: Allowed Infrequently	AVOID
Blackberry	Apricot	Apple	Currant	Banana
Blueberry	Boysen-	Asian pear	Date	Bitter melon
Cherry	berry	Avocado	Grape (all)	Coconut
Elderberry	Cranberry	Breadfruit	Pome-	Honeydew
(dark blue/	Fig (fresh/	Canang	granate	Mango
purple)	dried)	melon	Quince	Orange

SUPER BENEFICIAL	BENEFICIAL	NEUTRAL: Allowed Frequently	NEUTRAL: Allowed Infrequently	AVOID
Plum	Grapefruit	Cantaloupe	Raisin	Papaya
Prune	Lemon	Casaba	Star fruit	Plantain
	Lime	melon	(caram-	Tangerine
	Pineapple	Christmas	bola)	
		melon	Strawberry	
		Cranberry		
		(juice)		
		Crenshaw		
		melon		
		Dewberry		
		Gooseberry		
		Guava		
		Kiwi		
		Kumquat		
		Loganberry		
		Mulberry		
		Muskmelon		
		Nectarine		
		Peach		
		Pear		
		Persian		
		melon		
		Persimmon		
		Prickly pear		
		Raspberry		
		Sago palm		

SUPER BENEFICIAL	BENEFICIAL	NEUTRAL: Allowed Frequently	NEUTRAL: Allowed Infrequently	AVOID
		Spanish melon		
		Watermelon		
		Youngberry		

Special Variants: *Non-Secretor:* BENEFICIAL: cranberry (juice), elderberry (dark blue/purple), watermelon; NEUTRAL (Allowed Frequently): banana, coconut, lime, mango, plantain, tangerine; AVOID: cantaloupe, casaba melon.

Spices/Condiments/Sweeteners

Many spices have medicinal properties. Turmeric activates an enzyme that prevents oxidation in the brain. Garlic is a super antioxidant that minimizes inflammation and helps prevent neurological disease. Ginger contains an antioxidant called zingerone, which appears to have brain-protective properties. Many common food additives, such as guar gum and carrageenan, enhance the effects of lectins found in other foods and should be avoided.

SUPER BENEFICIAL	BENEFICIAL	NEUTRAL: Allowed Frequently	NEUTRAL: Allowed Infrequently	AVOID
Garlic	Barley malt	Agar	Brown rice syrup	Aspartame
Ginger	Coriander seeds	Allspice	Chocolate	Capers
Turmeric				Carrageenan

SUPER BENEFICIAL	BENEFICIAL	NEUTRAL: Allowed Frequently	NEUTRAL: Allowed Infrequently	AVOID
	Fenugreek	Almond	Cornstarch	Chili powder
	Horse-	extract	Corn syrup	Gelatin
	radish	Anise	Dextrose	(except
	Molasses	Apple pectin	Fructose	veg-
	(black-	Arrowroot	Guarana	sourced)
	strap)	Basil	Honey	Gums
	Mustard	Bay leaf	Malto-	(acacia/
	(dry)	Bergamot	dextrin	Arabic/
	Parsley	Caraway	Maple	guar)
	Soy sauce	Cardamon	syrup	Juniper
	Tamari	Carob	Rice syrup	Ketchup
	(wheat-	Chervil	Senna	Mayonnaise
	free)	Chive	Sugar	MSG
		Cilantro	(brown/	Pepper
		(coriander	white)	(black/
		leaf)		white)
		Cinnamon		Pepper
		Clove		(cayenne)
		Cream of		Pepper
		tartar		(pepper-
		Cumin		corn/red
		Dill		flakes)
		Invert sugar		Pickles/
		Licorice root*		relish
		Mace		Sucanat
		Marjoram		Vinegar (all)
		Mint (all)		Wintergreen

SUPER BENEFICIAL	BENEFICIAL	NEUTRAL: Allowed Frequently	NEUTRAL: Allowed Infrequently	AVOID
		Molasses		Worcester-
		Nutmeg		shire
		Oregano		sauce
		Paprika		
		Rosemary		
		Saffron		
		Sage		
		Savory		
		Sea salt		
		Seaweed		
		Stevia		
		Tamarind		
		Tarragon		
		Thyme		
		Vanilla		
		Vegetable glycerine		
		Yeast (baker's/ brewer's)		

Special Variants: *Non-Secretor:* BENEFICIAL: cilantro (coriander leaf), yeast (brewer's); NEUTRAL (Allowed Frequently): barley malt, chili powder, rice syrup, parsley, soy sauce, tamari (wheat-free), turmeric, wintergreen; AVOID: agar, cornstarch, corn syrup, dextrose, invert sugar, maltodextrin, senna.

* Do not use if you have high blood pressure.

Herbal Teas

Herbal teas can provide health benefits for Blood Type A. SUPER BENEFICIAL are chamomile and holy basil, which can reduce stress; dandelion and ginger, which aid digestion; and echinacea and rosehip, which can support immune health.

SUPER BENEFICIAL	BENEFICIAL	NEUTRAL: Allowed Frequently	NEUTRAL: Allowed Infrequently	AVOID
Chamomile	Alfalfa	Chickweed	Hops	Catnip
Dandelion	Aloe	Coltsfoot	Senna	Cayenne
Echinacea	Burdock	Dong quai		Corn silk
Ginger	Fenugreek	Elderberry		Red clover
Holy basil	Gentian	Goldenseal		Rhubarb
Rosehip	Ginkgo	Horehound		Yellow dock
	biloba	Licorice root*		
	Ginseng	Linden		
	Hawthorn	Mulberry		
	Milk thistle	Mullein		
	Parsley	Peppermint		
	Slippery	Raspberry		
	elm	leaf		
	St. John's	Sage		
	wort	Sarsaparilla		
	Stone root	Shepherd's		
	Valerian	purse		
		Skullcap		
		Spearmint		

SUPER BENEFICIAL	BENEFICIAL	NEUTRAL: Allowed Frequently	NEUTRAL: Allowed Infrequently	AVOID
		Strawberry leaf Thyme White birch White oak bark Yarrow		

Special Variants: *Non-Secretor:* AVOID: senna.

* Do not use if you have high blood pressure.

Miscellaneous Beverages

Green tea is a SUPER BENEFICIAL beverage for Blood Type A because it improves intracellular energy production. Red wine contains gallic acid, trans-resveratrol, quercetin, and rutin—four phenolic compounds with potent antioxidant effects. Blood Type A individuals who are not caffeine sensitive might consider having one cup of coffee daily; it contains many enzymes also found in soy, which can help the immune system function more effectively.

SUPER BENEFICIAL	BENEFICIAL	NEUTRAL: Allowed Frequently	NEUTRAL: Allowed Infrequently	AVOID
Tea (green)	Coffee (reg) Wine (red)	Coffee (decaf) Wine (white)		Beer Liquor Seltzer Soda (club) Soda (cola/ diet/ misc.) Tea, black (reg/ decaf)

Special Variants: *Non-Secretor:* BENEFICIAL: wine (white); NEUTRAL (Allowed Frequently): beer, seltzer, soda (club), tea (black: (reg/decaf).

Supplements

THE BLOOD TYPE A DIET offers abundant quantities of important nutrients, such as protein and iron. However, properly calibrated supplements can provide important benefits. This may be especially true as we age. Recent clinical studies showed that dietary supplements can treat nutritional deficiencies in the elderly, boost their immune systems, combat short-term memory loss, reduce risks of Alzheimer's, and improve seniors' overall health. The following supplement protocols are designed for Blood Type A individuals to improve brain health, cognitive function, and cellular integrity.

Note: if you are being treated for a medical condition, consult your doctor before taking any supplements.

Blood Type A: Basic Anti-Aging Protocol

Use this protocol 4–8 weeks, then discontinue for 2 weeks and restart.		
SUPPLEMENT	ACTION	DOSAGE
High-potency vitamin-mineral complex (preferably blood type–specific)	Nutritional support	As directed
N-acetyl cysteine (NAC)	A potent antioxidant, chelating agent, and the precursor of one of the body's primary protective agents, glutathione	100 mg, 1 capsule, 3 times daily
Betaine hydrochloride	Increases stomach acid; reduces stress; promotes healthy liver function and cellular energy	250 mg, 1 capsule with large meals
Plant enzyme formula	Helps break down foods into smaller, absorbable units for easier digestion	Formula contains: Lipase (20–25 mg capsule) Protease (20–25 mg capsule) Amylase (20–30 mg capsule) Rennin (5–10 mg capsule)

SUPPLEMENT	ACTION	DOSAGE
Probiotic (preferably blood type–specific)	Promotes intestinal health	1–2 capsules, twice daily
Sprouted food complex	Helps metabolize toxins and carcinogens; contains anti-inflammatory enzymes	2–3 capsules daily, preferably from Blood Type A–friendly food sources

Blood Type A:
Cognitive Improvement Protocol

Use this protocol 4–8 weeks, then discontinue for 2 weeks and restart.		
SUPPLEMENT	ACTION	DOSAGE
Brahmi (*Bacopa monnieri*)	Helps improve memory	200 mg, 1–2 capsules daily
OPCs (oligomeric proanthrocyandins)	Promotes intestinal health	100 mg, 1 capsule daily
Methylcobalamin (active vitamin B$_{12}$)	Plays important role in homocysteine regulation, red blood cell production, and maintaining nerve integrity	500 mcg daily

SUPPLEMENT	ACTION	DOSAGE
Spreading hogweed (*Boerhaavia diffusa*)	Has a dramatic effect in buffering against elevation of plasma cortisol levels under stressful conditions; acts to reverse the depletion of adrenal cortisol associated with adrenal exhaustion	50 mg, 1–2 capsules, twice daily
DHA (docosahexaenoic acid)	Omega-3 fatty acid, which provides fuel for brain metabolism and helps control inflammation	100 mg, 1 capsule daily

Blood Type A:
Immune System Health Protocol

Use this protocol for 4–8 weeks, then discontinue for 2 weeks and restart.		
SUPPLEMENT	ACTION	DOSAGE
Milk thistle (*Silymarin*)	Not only prevents the depletion of glutathione induced by alcohol and other toxic chemicals but has been shown	1–2 capsules, standardized extract, twice daily; try to take milk thistle with a meal containing

SUPPLEMENT	ACTION	DOSAGE
	to increase the level of glutathione	eggs, as studies have shown that when milk thistle is combined with phosphatidyl choline (found in eggs) its absorption is significantly higher.
Selenium	Mineral cofactor in the manufacture of glutathione peroxidase	50–100 mcg daily
Quercetin	Promotes digestive and intestinal integrity; controls inflammation; modulates allergic activity	200–500 mg, twice daily
Siberian ginseng (*Eleutherococcus senticosus*)	Increases resistance to stress and aids in recovery, thus reducing adrenal and thymic atrophy	100 mg, twice daily with meals

Blood Type A: Cellular Health Protocol

Use this protocol for 4–8 weeks, then discontinue for 2 weeks and restart.

SUPPLEMENT	ACTION	DOSAGE
Pantethine	Deficiency of this nutrient or its pantothenic acid, results in a decrease in adrenal function with the most noted symptom being fatigue; evidence indicates that supplementation normalizes the adrenal glands' capacity to respond to stress; may have beneficial effect in managing elevated cholesterol	500 mg, twice daily
Malic acid	Naturally occurring compound that plays a role in the complex process of deriving adenosine triphosphate (ATP), the energy currency that runs the body, from food	1,000 mg daily

SUPPLEMENT	ACTION	DOSAGE
Green tea	Improves cardio-vascular and immune health; contains xanthines, which are important facilitators of intracellular energy production	1–3 cups daily

The Exercise Component

FOR BLOOD TYPE A, overall fitness and immune health depend on engaging in regular exercises, with an emphasis on calming exercises such as hatha yoga and T'ai Chi, as well as light aerobic exercise such as walking.

The following comprises the ideal exercise regimen for Blood Type A:

EXERCISE	DURATION	FREQUENCY
Hatha yoga	40–50 minutes	3–4 x week
T'ai Chi	40–50 minutes	3–4 x week
Aerobics (low impact)	40–50 minutes	2–3 x week
Treadmill	30 minutes	2–3 x week
Pilates	40–50 minutes	3–4 x week
Weight training (5–10 lb free weights)	15 minutes	2–3 x week

EXERCISE	DURATION	FREQUENCY
Cycling (recumbent bike)	30 minutes	2–3 x week
Swimming	30 minutes	2–3 x week
Brisk walking	45 minutes	2–3 x week

3 Steps to Effective Exercise

1. Warm up with stretching and flexibility moves before you start your aerobic exercise.

2. To achieve maximum cardiovascular benefits, work toward an elevated heart rate that is about 70 percent of your capacity. Once you reach the elevated rate, continue exercising to maintain that rate for twenty to thirty minutes. To calculate your maximum heart rate and performance level:
   • Subtract your age from 220.
   • Multiply the difference by .70 (or .60 if you are over age sixty). This is the high end of your performance.
   • Multiply the remainder by .50. This is the low end of your performance.

3. Finish each aerobic session with at least a five-minute cooldown of stretching and relaxation moves.

Getting Started: The First Month

IF YOU ARE NEW to the Blood Type Diet, the following guidelines will introduce you to the Blood Type A regimen over a period of one month. Follow these recommendations as closely as possible, using a notebook to record your personal experiences with the diet. In addition to factors that are measurable in laboratory tests, take the time to note changes in your energy levels, sleep patterns, digestion, and overall well-being.

Blood Type A Brain-Boosting Diet Checklist

Avoid or limit animal proteins. Low levels of hydrochloric acid and intestinal alkaline phosphatase make them hard for Blood Type A to digest. ☐

Derive your primary protein from plant foods with seafood used occasionally. ☐

Seafood should be primarily richly oiled cold-water fish. ☐

Include modest amounts of cultured dairy foods in your diet, but avoid fresh milk products. ☐

Don't overdo the grains, especially wheat-derived foods. ☐

Eat lots of BENEFICIAL fruits and vegetables, especially those high in antioxidants and fiber. ☐

Drink green tea every day for extra immune system benefits. ☐

Week 1

Blood Type Diet and Supplements

- Eliminate your most harmful AVOID foods—red meat, most dairy, and negative lectin-containing nuts, beans, and seeds.
- Include your most important BENEFICIAL foods frequently throughout the week. For example, have soy-based foods 5 times, and omega-3-rich fish 3 to 4 times, with lots of BENEFICIAL vegetables and fruit.
- Incorporate at least 1 SUPER BENEFICIAL into your daily diet. For example, have a bowl of cherries as a snack, or a spinach salad with walnuts.
- If you have allergies, avoid whole-wheat products.
- Drink 2 to 3 cups of green tea every day.

Exercise Regimen

- Plan to exercise at least 4 days this week, for 45 minutes each day.
  2 days: walking or light aerobic activity
  2 days: yoga or T'ai Chi
- If you are ill or have low energy, start slowly and gradually increase your duration and intensity of activity. The important factor is consistency. Just do it—as much as you're able.
- Use your journal to detail the time, activity, and distance. Note the number of repetitions for each exercise.

■ WEEK 1 SUCCESS STRATEGY ■
Soothe and Strengthen Your Mind with Chi Breathing

Chi breathing is based upon the Taoist concept of Chi (Qi) Gong, which represents energy as flowing according to certain routes in your body. Positive release is accessible through refining the breath. The calming, stress-relieving effects of this exercise are remarkable. It can be performed by anyone, regardless of age, fitness, or medical condition.

1. Stand comfortably, feet shoulder-width apart, knees slightly bent, arms at your side. Relax your neck and shoulder muscles and focus on your solar plexus (center of the body). It is okay to sway a bit—that's normal.

2. Start to rock back and forth gently. Inhale deeply as you rock forward onto the balls of your feet; exhale as you rock backward onto your heels.

3. As you inhale, lift your relaxed arms up and forward, keeping them relaxed and slightly bent. As you exhale, let your arms float down. Imagine that your hands are pulsing around an imaginary ball of energy.

4. Repeat, gradually refining the rhythm and developing the ability to "drop" your breath from the lungs to the solar plexus.

5. Repeat four to five times, then relax, letting your hands drop to your sides and closing your eyes. Concentrate on feeling relaxed and centered.

Week 2

Blood Type Diet and Supplements

- Begin to eliminate the next level of AVOID foods—grains, vegetables, and fruits that react poorly with Type A blood.
- Eat 2 to 3 BENEFICIAL proteins every day, with special emphasis on soy. Eat omega-3-rich fish at least 3 times a week.
- Continue to incorporate SUPER BENEFICIAL foods into your daily diet.
- Choose the NEUTRAL foods listed as "Allowed Frequently" over those listed "Allowed Infrequently."
- Manage your mealtimes to aid proper digestion. Avoid eating on the run. Make your meals relaxing, sit-down affairs. Eat slowly and chew thoroughly to encourage digestive secretions.

Exercise Regimen

- Continue to exercise at least 4 days this week, for 45 minutes each day.
  2 days: walking or light aerobic activity
  2 days: yoga or T'ai Chi
- If your work is sedentary, get in the habit of taking a couple of "movement" breaks during the day. Walk around the block or up and down stairs.

■ WEEK 2 SUCCESS STRATEGY ■
Blood Type A Berry Brain Booster

Tufts University published a study involving several antioxidant-rich extracts such as spinach and blueberries. While all scored well in enhancing memory improvement, only blueberries had a significant impact on improving motor skills like balance and coordination. While previous research has indicated that antioxidants may help lower the risk of cancer and heart disease, these new findings are the first to reveal a connection between potent antioxidants like blueberries and age-related declines. How do blueberries work? The authors of the Tufts study theorize that because blueberries keep the cell membranes healthy, they allow for more effective transport of important nutrients.

Blend together:

1 cup mixed berries (blueberries, blackberries, elderberries)

1 cup light soy milk*

ice

*If desired, substitute Protein Blend 4 A, available through www.dadamo.com.

Week 3

Blood Type Diet and Supplements

- When you plan your meals for week 3, choose BENEFICIAL foods to replace NEUTRAL foods whenever possible. For example, choose tofu over chicken, or blueberries over an apple.
- Eliminate all remaining AVOID foods.
- Liberally incorporate SUPER BENEFICIAL foods into your daily diet.
- Drink 2 or 3 cups of green tea every day.

Exercise Regimen

- Continue to exercise at least 4 days this week, for 45 minutes each day.
  2 days: walking or light aerobic activity
  2 days: yoga or T'ai Chi

▪ WEEK 3 SUCCESS STRATEGY ▪
Rest Your Brain

Studies show that not getting enough sleep can have a drastic effect on cognitive function. For Type A, high cortisol levels can disrupt your sleep cycle, and you may have to work harder to get a good night's sleep. Try to establish a regular sleep schedule and adhere to it as closely as possible. When you have a normal sleep-wake rhythm, it reduces cortisol levels. During the day, schedule at least two breaks of twenty minutes each for complete relaxation. Combat sleep disturbances with regular exercise and a relaxing pre-bedtime routine. A light snack before bedtime will help raise your blood sugar levels and improve sleep.

If these strategies don't work, ask your doctor about the following supplement:

Methylcobalamin (active vitamin B₁₂): 1 3 mg per day taken in the morning. This vitamin enables deep sleep and helps you wake feeling more rested. Methylcobalamin also helps folic acid lower homocysteine.

Week 4

Blood Type Diet and Supplements

- Continue at the week 3 level, focusing on BENEFICIAL and SUPER BENEFICIAL foods.

Exercise Regimen

- Continue at the week 3 level.
- Review your progress, noting in your journal improvements in strength and flexibility. Determine which exercise regimen has worked for you, including time of day, setting, and activity level.

■ **WEEK 4 SUCCESS STRATEGY** ■
Maximize Energy with the Right Eating Schedule

For Blood Type A, the timing of your meals can be almost as important as what you eat. This is particularly true if you're trying to lose weight. The following are helpful guidelines:

- Never skip meals. You won't be "saving" calories, as the metabolic reaction will foil your efforts.
- Make breakfast your most important protein-rich meal of the day. The result will be an efficient metabolism all day long.
- Eat on a sliding scale: big breakfast, medium lunch, small dinner.
- Resist the late-night munchies, but if you have problems regulating blood sugar, have a small protein snack—yogurt or soy milk—before bedtime.

Blood Type

B

BLOOD TYPE B DIET OUTCOME: THREE-DAY MIRACLE

"Three days. It took only three days on the Type B Diet before I noticed a significant change. Two days later my coworkers started saying they noticed changes. My hair is growing back in after thirteen years of thinning. My short-term memory is improving over time. My back is stronger, due to exercise, diet, and increased energy."

Self-reported outcome from the Blood Type Diet Web site
(www.dadamo.com).

Blood Type B: The Foods

THE BLOOD TYPE B Fight Aging Diet is specifically adapted to provide the maximum nutritional support to fight many of the conditions associated with aging. A new

Aurora Public Library

(905)-727-9494

www.aurorapl.ca

Checked Out Items 27/08/2018 18:16
23164001393369

Item Title	Due Date
33164300207508	17/09/2018
Aging : fight it with the blood diet	
33164100059315	/2018
Divergent	

category, **Super Beneficial**, highlights powerful disease-fighting foods for Blood Type B. The **Neutral** category has also been adjusted to de-emphasize foods that are less advantageous for you. Foods designated **Neutral: Allowed Infrequently** should be minimized or avoided entirely.

Your secretor status can influence your ability to fully digest and metabolize certain foods, so various adjustments in the values are made for non-secretors. If you do not know your secretor type, the odds are that you can safely use the "secretor" values, since the majority of the population (approximately 80 percent) are secretors. However, I urge you to get tested, since the variations are important for non-secretors who want to maximize the effectiveness of the Blood Type Diet.

Blood Type B

TOP 12 BRAIN POWER SUPER FOODS

1. lean, organic, grass-fed red meat (especially lamb or mutton)
2. richly oiled cold-water fish (halibut, sardines)
3. cultured dairy (kefir, yogurt)
4. olive oil
5. walnuts
6. maitake/shiitake mushrooms
7. beets
8. greens (collard, kale)
9. berries (cranberry, elderberry)
10. watermelon
11. ginseng tea
12. green tea

The food charts are divided into three sections. The top of the chart suggests the average portion size and quantity per week or day, according to secretor status. These recommendations do *not* apply to the category **Neutral: Allowed Infrequently**; those foods should be eaten rarely, if at all. The charts also indicate differences in frequency for some foods, based on ethnic heritage. It has been my experience that this factor has an impact upon the individual's ability to fully digest certain foods. For the purposes of blood type food choices, persons of Hispanic heritage should follow the guidelines for Caucasians, and American Native peoples should follow the guidelines for Asians.

The middle section of the chart gives the food values. The bottom section lists variants based on secretor status.

For your convenience, we have included a number of product names (Ezekiel 4:9 bread, Worcestershire sauce, etc.). However, keep in mind that commercial formulations vary among brands and regions. For example, there are several forms of Ezekiel 4:9 bread, and not all may be right for your type. Even though a product may be listed as acceptable for you, always check its ingredients. Some products contain **Avoid** ingredients for your blood type. Of course, you may choose to make your own version of commercial products, such as bread and mayonnaise, using ingredients that suit your blood type. There are hundreds of delicious recipes for every blood type available on our Web site (www.dadamo.com) and in the book *Cook Right 4 Your Type: The Practical Kitchen Companion to* Eat Right 4 Your Type.

Meat/Poultry

Blood Type B is able to efficiently metabolize animal protein, but there are limitations that require careful dietary navigation. Chicken, one of the most popular food choices, disagrees with Blood Type B because of a B-specific agglutinin, called a galectin, contained in the organ and muscle meat. This galectin can trigger inflammatory and autoimmune conditions. Turkey does not contain this lectin and can be eaten as an excellent alternative to chicken. Choose only the best quality (preferably free-range) chemical-, antibiotic-, and pesticide-free low-fat meats and poultry. Grass-fed cattle are far superior to grain-fed.

BLOOD TYPE B: MEATS/POULTRY
Portion: 4–6 oz (men); 2–5 oz (women and children)

	African	Caucasian	Asian
Secretor	3–6	2–6	2–5
Non-Secretor	4–7	4–7	4–7
		Times per week	

SUPER BENEFICIAL	BENEFICIAL	NEUTRAL: Allowed Frequently	NEUTRAL: Allowed Infrequently	AVOID
Goat	Rabbit	Beef		All commercially
Lamb	Venison	Buffalo		processed
Mutton		Liver (calf)		meats
		Ostrich		Bacon/ham/
		Pheasant		pork
		Turkey		Chicken
		Veal		Cornish hen

SUPER BENEFICIAL	BENEFICIAL	NEUTRAL: Allowed Frequently	NEUTRAL: Allowed Infrequently	AVOID
				Duck
				Goose
				Grouse
				Guinea hen
				Heart (beef)
				Horse
				Partridge
				Quail
				Squab
				Squirrel
				Sweetbreads
				Turtle

Special Variants: *Non-Secretor:* BENEFICIAL: liver (calf); NEUTRAL (Allowed Frequently): heart (beef), horse, squab, sweetbreads.

Fish/Seafood

Richly oiled cold-water fish, such as halibut, mackerel, cod, salmon, and sardines, are especially good protein sources for Type B, since they are excellent sources of omega-3 fatty acids and the essential fatty acids EPA and DHA, which provide fuel for brain metabolism and help control inflammation. Salmon, halibut, and sardines are good sources of phosphorus, needed for energy production. Caviar (sturgeon) is an excellent source of very long-chain fatty acids, vitamins A and D, and zinc.

BLOOD TYPE B: FISH/SEAFOOD
Portion: 4–6 oz (men); 2–5 oz (women and children)

	African	Caucasian	Asian
Secretor	4–5	3–5	3–5
Non-Secretor	4–5	4–5	4–5
	Times per week		

SUPER BENEFICIAL	BENEFICIAL	NEUTRAL: Allowed Frequently	NEUTRAL: Allowed Infrequently	AVOID
Caviar (sturgeon)	Croaker	Abalone	Herring (pickled/ smoked)	Anchovy
Cod	Flounder	Bluefish	Salmon (smoked)	Barracuda
Halibut	Grouper	Bullhead	Scallops	Bass (all)
Mackerel	Haddock	Carp		Beluga
Salmon (caught, not farm raised)	Hake	Catfish		Butterfish
Sardine	Harvest fish	Chub		Clam
	Mahimahi	Cusk		Conch
	Monkfish	Drum		Crab
	Perch (ocean)	Gray sole		Crayfish
	Pickerel	Halfmoon fish		Eel
	Pike	Herring (fresh)		Frog
	Porgy	Mullet		Lobster
	Shad	Muskellunge		Mussel
	Sole	Opaleye		Octopus
	Sturgeon	Orange roughy		Oysters
		Parrot fish		Pollock
				Shrimp

SUPER BENEFICIAL	BENEFICIAL	NEUTRAL: Allowed Frequently	NEUTRAL: Allowed Infrequently	AVOID
		Perch (silver/ white/ yellow)		Snail (*Helix pomatia/ escargot*)
		Pompano		Trout (all)
		Red snapper		Yellowtail
		Rosefish		
		Sailfish		
		Scrod		
		Scup		
		Shark		
		Smelt		
		Sole (gray)		
		Squid (cala-mari)		
		Sucker		
		Sunfish		
		Swordfish		
		Tilapia		
		Tilefish		
		Tuna		
		Weakfish		
		Whitefish		
		Whiting		

Special Variants: *Non-Secretor:* BENEFICIAL: carp; NEUTRAL (Allowed Frequently): barracuda, butterfish, caviar (sturgeon), flounder, halibut, pike, salmon, gray sole, snail (*Helix pomatia/escargot*), yellowtail; AVOID: scallops.

Dairy/Eggs

Dairy products, especially cultured dairy products, can be eaten by almost all Blood Type B secretors, and to a lesser degree by non-secretors. Cultured dairy, such as yogurt and kefir, is particularly good for Blood Type B; these foods help build a healthy intestinal environment. Kefir has been studied for its role in improving the oxygen supply to the brain. Yogurt is a good source of pantothenic acid, a B vitamin essential for energy metabolism and cognitive function. The lactic acid in whole buttermilk has a beneficial effect in optimizing blood flow through the carotid arteries. Eggs can be eaten in moderation. They are an excellent source of DHA and contain choline, which increases energy and enhances memory. Ghee (clarified butter) contains BENEFICIAL fatty acids believed to promote intestinal balance. Non-secretors should be wary of eating too much cheese, as they are more sensitive to many of the microbial strains in aged cheeses. This sensitivity is greater for those of African ancestry, but the sensitivity can also be found in Caucasian and Asian populations. Cheese consumption should also be limited for those who suffer from recurrent infections or allergies, as cheese can trigger inflammation and produce excess mucus. Do your best to find dairy products that are both hormone-free and organic.

BLOOD TYPE B: EGGS Portion: 1 egg			
	African	**Caucasian**	**Asian**
Secretor	3–4	3–4	3–4
Non-Secretor	5–6	5–6	5–6
		Times per week	

BLOOD TYPE B: MILK AND YOGURT
Portion: 4–6 oz (men); 2–5 oz (women and children)

	African	Caucasian	Asian
Secretor	3–5	3–4	3–4
Non-Secretor	1–3	2–4	1–3
		Times per week	

BLOOD TYPE B: CHEESE
Portion: 3 oz (men); 2 oz (women and children)

	African	Caucasian	Asian
Secretor	3–4	3–5	3–4
Non-Secretor	1–4	1–4	1–4
		Times per week	

SUPER BENEFICIAL	BENEFICIAL	NEUTRAL: Allowed Frequently	NEUTRAL: Allowed Infrequently	AVOID
Buttermilk	Cottage	Camembert	Brie	American
Ghee	cheese	Casein	Butter	cheese
(clarified	Farmer	Cream	Cheddar	Blue cheese
butter)	cheese	cheese	Colby	Egg (duck/
Kefir	Feta	Edam	Half-and-	goose/
Yogurt	Goat	Egg (chicken)	half	quail)
	cheese	Emmenthal	Jarlsberg	Ice cream
	Milk (cow/	Gouda	Monterey	
	goat)	Gruyère	Jack	
			Muenster	

SUPER BENEFICIAL	BENEFICIAL	NEUTRAL: Allowed Frequently	NEUTRAL: Allowed Infrequently	AVOID
	Mozzarella Paneer Ricotta	Neufchâtel Parmesan Provolone Quark Sour cream	Sherbet Swiss cheese Whey	

Special Variants: *Non-Secretor:* BENEFICIAL: whey; NEUTRAL (Allowed Frequently): cottage cheese, milk (cow); AVOID: Camembert, cheddar, Emmenthal, Jarlsberg, Monterey Jack, Muenster, Parmesan, provolone, Swiss cheese.

Oils

Blood Type B does best on monounsaturated oils and oils rich in omega series fatty acids. Olive oil fits the bill in both regards and should be used as the primary cooking oil. Constituents in olive oil, such as flavonoids, squalenes, and polyphenols, act as powerful antioxidants. Flax (linseed) oil is high in alpha-linolenic acid, which aids brain cell connectivity.

Sesame, sunflower, and corn oils should be avoided as they contain immunoreactive proteins that impair Blood Type B digestion.

BLOOD TYPE B: OILS
Portion: 1 tblsp

	African	Caucasian	Asian
Secretor	5–8	5–8	5–8
Non-Secretor	3–5	3–7	3–6
		Times per week	

SUPER BENEFICIAL	BENEFICIAL	NEUTRAL: Allowed Frequently	NEUTRAL: Allowed Infrequently	AVOID
Flax (linseed) Olive		Almond Black currant seed Cod liver Evening primrose Walnut	Wheat germ	Avocado Canola Castor Coconut Corn Cottonseed Peanut Safflower Sesame Soy Sunflower

Special Variants: *Non-Secretor:* BENEFICIAL: black currant seed, walnut.

Nuts/Seeds

Nuts and seeds can be an important secondary source of protein for Blood Type B. Walnuts are highly effective in inhibiting gastrointestinal toxicity; raw flaxseeds contain BENEFICIAL immunity-enhancing chemicals. As with other aspects of the Blood Type B Diet plan, there are some idiosyncratic elements to the choice of seeds and nuts: Several, such as sunflower and sesame, have B-agglutinating lectins and should be avoided.

BLOOD TYPE B: NUTS/SEEDS
Portion: Whole (handful); Nut Butters (2 tblsp)

	African	Caucasian	Asian
Secretor	4–7	4–7	4–7
Non-Secretor	5–7	5–7	5–7
	Times per week		

SUPER BENEFICIAL	BENEFICIAL	NEUTRAL: Allowed Frequently	NEUTRAL: Allowed Infrequently	AVOID
Flax (linseed)		Almond	Lychee	Cashew
Walnut (black)		Almond butter	Macadamia	Filbert (hazelnut)
		Beechnut	Pecan	Peanut
		Brazil nut		Peanut butter
		Butternut		Pignolia (pine nut)
		Chestnut		Pistachio
		Hickory		Poppy seed
		Walnut (English)		Pumpkin seed

SUPER BENEFICIAL	BENEFICIAL	NEUTRAL: Allowed Frequently	NEUTRAL: Allowed Infrequently	AVOID
				Safflower seed Sesame butter (tahini) Sesame seed Sunflower seed

Special Variants: *Non-Secretor:* BENEFICIAL: walnut (English); NEUTRAL (Allowed Frequently): pumpkin seed.

Beans and Legumes

Blood Type B can do well on the proteins found in many beans and legumes, although this food category does contain more than a few beans with problematic lectins. Soy products should be de-emphasized, as they are rich in a class of enzymes that can interact negatively with the B antigen. Several beans, such as mung beans, contain B-agglutinating lectins and should be avoided.

BLOOD TYPE B: BEANS AND LEGUMES
Portion: 1 cup cooked

	African	Caucasian	Asian
Secretor	5–7	5–7	5–7
Non-Secretor	3–5	3–5	3–5
		Times per week	

SUPER BENEFICIAL	BENEFICIAL	NEUTRAL: Allowed Frequently	NEUTRAL: Allowed Infrequently	AVOID
	Bean (green/ snap/ string)	Cannellini bean	Soy bean	Adzuki bean
	Fava (broad) bean	Copper bean		Black bean
	Kidney bean	Jicama bean		Black-eyed pea
	Lima bean	Pea (green/ pod/snow)		Garbanzo (chickpea)
	Navy bean	Tamarind bean		Lentil (all)
	Northern bean	White bean		Mung bean/ sprouts
				Pinto bean
				Soy cheese
				Soy milk
				Soy, miso
				Soy, tempeh
				Soy, tofu

Special Variants: *Non-Secretor:* NEUTRAL (Allowed Frequently): bean (green/snap/string), fava (broad) bean, kidney bean, lima bean, navy bean, northern bean, soy milk; AVOID: soy bean.

Grains and Starches

Grains are a leading factor in triggering inflammatory and autoimmune conditions in Blood Type B. The wheat agglutinin is particularly harmful, as is the lectin in corn. Non-secretors have an even greater sensitivity to these lectins. Wheat sensitivity has been linked to neurological and behavioral problems. Sprouted grains, such as Essene bread (manna), are the exception. Sprouting makes the grains less reactive to the Type B immune system.

BLOOD TYPE B: GRAINS AND STARCHES
Portion: ¼ cup dry (grains or pastas); 1 muffin; 2 slices of bread

	African	Caucasian	Asian
Secretor	5–7	5–9	5–9
Non-Secretor	3–5	3–5	3–5
		Times per week	

SUPER BENEFICIAL	BENEFICIAL	NEUTRAL: Allowed Frequently	NEUTRAL: Allowed Infrequently	AVOID
	Essene bread (manna) Ezekiel 4:9 bread Millet Oat bran Oat flour	Barley Quinoa Spelt flour/ products	Rice flour Soy flour/ products Wheat (refined/ un-bleached)	Amaranth Buckwheat Cornmeal Couscous Grits Kamut Popcorn

SUPER BENEFICIAL	BENEFICIAL	NEUTRAL: Allowed Frequently	NEUTRAL: Allowed Infrequently	AVOID
	Oatmeal		Wheat (semolina)	Rice (wild)
	Rice bran		Wheat (white flour)	Rye
	Rice cake			Rye flour
	Rice milk			Soba noodles (100% buckwheat)
	Spelt (whole)			Sorghum
				Tapioca
				Teff
				Wheat (whole)
				Wheat bran
				Wheat germ

Special Variants: *Non-Secretor:* NEUTRAL (Allowed Frequently): amaranth, Ezekiel 4:9 bread, oat (all), rice (wild), sorghum, spelt (whole), tapioca; AVOID: soy flour/products, wheat (all).

Vegetables

Vegetables can be your first line of defense against chronic disease. They provide a rich source of antioxidants and fiber and are essential to intestinal health. SUPER BENEFICIAL vegetables, such as maitake and shiitake mushrooms, are rich sources of antioxidants and immune modulators. Cabbage, cauliflower, and Brussels sprouts reduce the production of toxins in the digestive tract. Onions and broccoli are potent detoxifiers. Broccoli contains allyl methyl trisulfide and dithiolthiones, which increase the activity of enzymes involved in detoxification.

Tomatoes contain a lectin that reacts with the saliva and digestive juices of Blood Type B secretors, although it does not appear to react with non-secretors. Corn has B-agglutinating activity and should be avoided.

An item's value also applies to its juice, unless otherwise noted.

BLOOD TYPE B: VEGETABLES
Portion: 1 cup, prepared (cooked or raw)

	African	Caucasian	Asian
Secretor Super/ Beneficials	Unlimited	Unlimited	Unlimited
Secretor Neutrals	2–5	2–5	2–5
Non-Secretor Super/Beneficials	Unlimited	Unlimited	Unlimited
Non-Secretor Neutrals	2–3	2–3	2–3
	Times per day		

SUPER BENEFICIAL	BENEFICIAL	NEUTRAL: Allowed Frequently	NEUTRAL: Allowed Infrequently	AVOID
Broccoli	Beet	Alfalfa	Potato	Aloe
Brussels sprouts	Beet greens	sprouts		Artichoke
	Carrot	Arugula		Corn

SUPER BENEFICIAL	BENEFICIAL	NEUTRAL: Allowed Frequently	NEUTRAL: Allowed Infrequently	AVOID
Cabbage	Collards	Asparagus		Olive (all)
Cabbage (juice)*	Eggplant	Asparagus pea		Pumpkin
Cauliflower	Kale	Bamboo shoots		Radish/ sprouts
Mushroom (maitake/ shiitake)	Mustard greens	Bok choy		Rhubarb
Onion (all)	Parsnip	Carrot (juice)		Tomato
	Peppers (all)	Celeriac		
	Potato (sweet)	Celery		
	Yam	Chicory		
		Cucumber		
		Daikon radish		
		Dandelion		
		Endive		
		Escarole		
		Fennel		
		Fiddlehead fern		
		Garlic		
		Horseradish		
		Kohlrabi		
		Leek		
		Lettuce (all)		

SUPER BENEFICIAL	BENEFICIAL	NEUTRAL: Allowed Frequently	NEUTRAL: Allowed Infrequently	AVOID
		Mushroom (abalone/ enoki/ oyster/ portobello/ silver dollar/ straw/tree ear)		
		Okra		
		Oyster plant		
		Pickle (in brine or vinegar)		
		Poi		
		Radicchio		
		Rappini (broccoli rabe)		
		Rutabaga		
		Scallion		
		Seaweed		
		Shallot		
		Spinach		
		Squash (all)		
		Swiss chard		
		Taro		

SUPER BENEFICIAL	BENEFICIAL	NEUTRAL: Allowed Frequently	NEUTRAL: Allowed Infrequently	AVOID
		Turnip		
		Water chestnut		
		Watercress		
		Yucca		
		Zucchini		

Special Variants: *Non-Secretor:* BENEFICIAL: okra, NEUTRAL (Allowed frequently): artichoke, cabbage, eggplant, peppers (all), pumpkin, tomato, AVOID: potato.

* To obtain the benefits of cabbage juice, it must be consumed within one minute of juicing.

Fruits and Fruit Juices

Many SUPER BENEFICIAL fruits have powerful antioxidant effects, which help to reduce infection. Elderberries are particularly effective against viral infections. Watermelon improves nitric oxide synthesis and reduces edema. Plums are high in the phytonutrients neochlorogenic and chlorogenic acids. These substances are classified as phenols, and their function as antioxidants has been well-documented. Cranberries are SUPER BENEFICIAL for Blood Type B individuals, especially non-secretors, who have a higher than average risk for urinary tract infections. Blueberries have been studied for their anti-aging and antioxidant properties.

An item's value also applies to its juice, unless otherwise noted.

BLOOD TYPE B: FRUITS AND FRUIT JUICES
Portion: 1 cup

	African	Caucasian	Asian
Secretor	2–4	3–5	3–5
Non-Secretor	2–3	2–3	2–3
	Times per day		

SUPER BENEFICIAL	BENEFICIAL	NEUTRAL: Allowed Frequently	NEUTRAL: Allowed Infrequently	AVOID
Blueberry	Banana	Apple	Apricot	Avocado
Cranberry	Grape	Blackberry	Asian pear	Bitter melon
Elderberry	Papaya	Blueberry	Breadfruit	Coconut
(dark	Pineapple	Boysenberry	Cantaloupe	Persimmon
blue/		Canang	Currant	Pome-
purple)		melon	Date	granate
Plum		Casaba	Fig (fresh/	Prickly pear
Watermelon		melon	dried)	Star fruit
		Cherry (all)	Honeydew	(caram-
		Christmas	Plantain	bola)
		melon	Raisin	
		Crenshaw		
		melon		
		Dewberry		
		Gooseberry		
		Grapefruit		
		Guava		
		Kiwi		
		Kumquat		

SUPER BENEFICIAL	BENEFICIAL	NEUTRAL: Allowed Frequently	NEUTRAL: Allowed Infrequently	AVOID
		Lemon		
		Lime		
		Loganberry		
		Mango		
		Mulberry		
		Muskmelon		
		Nectarine		
		Orange		
		Peach		
		Pear		
		Persian melon		
		Prune		
		Quince		
		Raspberry		
		Sago palm		
		Spanish melon		
		Strawberry		
		Tangerine		
		Youngberry		

Special Variants: *Non-Secretor:* BENEFICIAL: blackberry, blueberry, boysenberry, cherry, currant, elderberry (dark blue/purple), fig (fresh/dried), guava, raspberry; NEUTRAL (Allowed Frequently): banana; AVOID: cantaloupe, honeydew.

Spices and Condiments

Many spices are known to have medicinal properties. Turmeric activates an enzyme that prevents oxidation in the brain. Ginger contains an antioxidant called zingerone, which appears to have brain protective properties. Licorice provides antiviral support and is important in effectively processing cortisol. Cayenne pepper is anti-inflammatory. Many common food additives, such as guar gum and carrageenan, enhance the effects of lectins found in other foods and should be avoided. Use caution when using prepared condiments, as they often contain wheat.

SUPER BENEFICIAL	BENEFICIAL	NEUTRAL: Allowed Frequently	NEUTRAL: Allowed Infrequently	AVOID
Ginger	Horse-	Anise	Agar	Allspice
Licorice	radish	Apple pectin	Arrowroot	Almond
root*	Molasses	Basil	Chocolate	extract
Pepper	(black-	Bay leaf	Fructose	Aspartame
(cayenne)	strap)	Bergamot	Honey	Barley malt
Turmeric	Parsley	Caper	Maple syrup	Carrageenan
		Caraway	Mayonnaise	Cinnamon
		Cardamom	Molasses	Cornstarch
		Carob	Pickles (all)	Corn syrup
		Chervil	Rice syrup	Dextrose
		Chili powder	Sugar	Gelatin
		Chive	(brown/	(except
			white)	veg-
				sourced)

SUPER BENEFICIAL	BENEFICIAL	NEUTRAL: Allowed Frequently	NEUTRAL: Allowed Infrequently	AVOID
		Cilantro (coriander leaf)	Tamari (wheat-free)	Guarana
		Clove	Vinegar (all)	Gums (acacia/ Arabic/ guar)
		Coriander		Invert sugar
		Cream of tartar		Juniper
		Cumin		Ketchup
		Dill		Malto-dextrin
		Fenugreek		MSG
		Garlic		Pepper (black/ white)
		Lecithin		Soy sauce
		Mace		Stevia
		Marjoram		Sucanat
		Mint (all)		Tapioca
		Mustard (dry)		
		Nutmeg		
		Oregano		
		Paprika		
		Pepper (pep-percorn/ red flakes)		
		Rosemary		
		Saffron		
		Sage		
		Savory		
		Sea salt		

SUPER BENEFICIAL	BENEFICIAL	NEUTRAL: Allowed Frequently	NEUTRAL: Allowed Infrequently	AVOID
		Seaweed		
		Senna		
		Tamarind		
		Tarragon		
		Thyme		
		Vanilla		
		Wintergreen		
		Yeast (baker's/ brewer's)		

Special Variants: *Non-Secretor:* BENEFICIAL: oregano, yeast (brewer's); NEUTRAL (Allowed Frequently): stevia; AVOID: agar, fructose, pickle relish, sugar (brown/white).

* Do not use if you have high blood pressure.

Herbal Teas

Several herbal teas are SUPER BENEFICIAL for Blood Type B. Ginger contains pungent phenolic substances with pronounced antioxidative and anti-inflammatory activities. Ginseng is known for its ability to improve cognitive function and reduce stress. Licorice provides antiviral support and is important in effectively processing cortisol.

SUPER BENEFICIAL	BENEFICIAL	NEUTRAL: Allowed Frequently	NEUTRAL: Allowed Infrequently	AVOID
Ginger	Dandelion	Alfalfa	Dong quai	Aloe
Ginseng	Parsley	Burdock		Coltsfoot
Licorice root*	Peppermint	Catnip		Corn silk
	Raspberry leaf	Chamomile		Fenugreek
	Rosehip	Chickweed		Gentian
	Sage	Echinacea		Hops
		Elder		Linden
		Goldenseal		Mullein
		Hawthorn		Red clover
		Horehound		Rhubarb
		Mulberry		Shepherd's purse
		Rosemary		Skullcap
		Sarsaparilla		
		Senna		
		Slippery elm		
		Spearmint		
		St. John's wort		
		Strawberry leaf		
		Thyme		
		Valerian		
		Vervain		
		White birch		
		White oak bark		
		Yarrow		
		Yellow dock		

Special Variants: None.

*Do not use if you have high blood pressure.

Miscellaneous Beverages

Green tea should be part of every Blood Type B's health plan. It contains polyphenols, which enhance intracellular energy and improve gastrointestinal health. Alcohol can exacerbate autoimmune inflammatory conditions. Avoid or limit alcohol to an occasional glass of red wine. If you are a heavy coffee drinker, try to reduce your intake or slowly eliminate it altogether.

SUPER BENEFICIAL	BENEFICIAL	NEUTRAL: Allowed Frequently	NEUTRAL: Allowed Infrequently	AVOID
Tea (green)		Wine (red/ white)	Beer Coffee (reg/ decaf) Tea, black (reg/ decaf)	Liquor Seltzer Soda (club) Soda (cola/ diet/ misc.)

Special Variants: *Non-Secretor:* BENEFICIAL: wine (red/white); NEUTRAL (Allowed Frequently): liquor, seltzer, soda (club); AVOID: coffee (reg/decaf), tea, black (reg/decaf).

Supplements

THE BLOOD TYPE B DIET offers abundant quantities of important nutrients, such as protein and iron. However, properly calibrated supplements can provide important benefits, and this may be especially true as we age. Recent clinical studies showed that dietary supplements can treat nutritional deficiencies in the elderly, boost their immune systems, combat short-term memory loss, reduce risks of Alzheimer's, and improve seniors' overall health. The following supplement protocols are designed for Blood Type B individuals to improve brain health, cognitive function, and cellular integrity.

Note: If you are being treated for a medical condition, consult your doctor before taking any supplements.

Blood Type B: Basic Anti-Aging Protocol

Use this protocol for 4–8 weeks, then discontinue for 2 weeks and restart.

SUPPLEMENT	ACTION	DOSAGE
High-potency vitamin-mineral complex (preferably blood type–specific)	Nutritional support	As directed
Magnesium citrate	Essential for nerve and digestive health	250 mg, 2 capsules, twice daily
Vinpocetine	Experiments indicate that it can enhance circulation in the brain, improve oxygen utilization, make red blood cells more pliable, and inhibit aggregation of platelets	10 mg, twice daily

SUPPLEMENT	ACTION	DOSAGE
Siberian ginseng (*Eleutherococcus senticosus*)	Increases resistance to stress and aids in recovery, thus reducing adrenal and thymic atrophy	100 mg, twice daily with meals

Blood Type B:
Cognitive Improvement Protocol

Use this protocol for 4–8 weeks, then discontinue for 2 weeks and restart.		
SUPPLEMENT	ACTION	DOSAGE
Gokharu/Caltrop (*Tribulus terrestris*) fruit extract; 20% furanosterols	Improves strength and protection against infection	50 mg, 1–2 capsules daily
Ginko (*Ginkgo biloba*)	Improves blood flow to the brain and enhances memory	24% standardized extract, 60 mg, 1–2 capsules daily
Creatine monohydrate	May compensate for deficiencies in energy metabolism, which accompany neuro-degenerative diseases	3–6 g daily

Blood Type B:
Immune System Health Protocol

Use this protocol for 4–8 weeks, then discontinue for 2 weeks and restart.

SUPPLEMENT	ACTION	DOSAGE
Larch arabinogalactan	Promotes digestive and intestinal health	1 tablespoon, twice daily, in juice or water
Maitake extract (*Grifola frondosa*)	Improves immune function	500 mg, 2–3 capsules, twice daily
Carob (*Ceratonia siliqua*)	Useful for nervous exhaustion	Solid extract, ¼–½ teaspoon, twice daily
Eucommia bark (*Cortex eucommiae*)	Traditionally used in Chinese medicine for nourishing the liver and kidney and strengthening the bones and muscles	10–15 g, decocted in water, twice daily

Blood Type B: Cellular Health Protocol

Use this protocol for 4–8 weeks, then discontinue for 2 weeks and restart.

SUPPLEMENT	ACTION	DOSAGE
L-arginine	Facilitates immune function and increases nitric oxide synthesis	250 mg, 1–2 capsules, twice daily
Licorice (*Glycyrrhiza sp*)*	Supports liver function; licorice contains glycyrrhizin, which is absorbed as glycyrrhetinic acid; glycyrrhizin inhibits an enzyme called 11–beta–hydroxysteroid dehydrogenase, which converts cortisol to cortisone	1 cup of tea, twice daily, or herbal preparations under direction of a physician
Potassium citrate	Necessary for proper protein and carbohydrate metabolism; synergistic with licorice	99 mg,1 capsule, twice daily

*Licorice can cause sodium and water retention. It should be used with a potassium supplement or in conjunction with a high-potassium diet.

The Exercise Component

FOR BLOOD TYPE B, stress regulation and overall fitness are achieved with a balance of moderate aerobic activity and mentally soothing, stress-reducing exercises. Below is a list of exercises that are recommended for Blood Type B.

EXERCISE	DURATION	FREQUENCY
Tennis	45–60 minutes	2–3 x week
Martial arts	30–60 minutes	2–3 x week
Cycling	45–60 minutes	2–3 x week
Hiking	30–60 minutes	2–3 x week
Golf (no cart)	60–90 minutes	2–3 x week
Running or brisk walking	40–50 minutes	2–3 x week
Pilates	40–50 minutes	2–3 x week
Swimming	45 minutes	2–3 x week
Yoga	40–50 minutes	1–2 x week
T'ai Chi	40–50 minutes	1–2 x week

3 Steps to Effective Exercise

1. Warm up with stretching and flexibility moves before you start your aerobic exercise.

2. To achieve maximum cardiovascular benefits, work toward an elevated heart rate that is about 70 percent of your capacity. Once you reach the elevated rate, continue exercising to maintain that rate for twenty to thirty minutes. To calculate your maximum heart rate and performance level:
   - Subtract your age from 220.
   - Multiply the difference by .70 (or .60 if you are over age sixty). This is the high end of your performance.
   - Multiply the remainder by .50. This is the low end of your performance.

3. Finish each aerobic session with at least a five-minute cooldown of stretching and relaxation moves.

Getting Started: The First Month

IF YOU ARE NEW to the Blood Type Diet, the following guidelines will introduce you to the Blood Type B regimen over a period of one month. Follow these recommendations as closely as possible, using a notebook to record your personal experiences with the diet. In addition to factors that are measurable in laboratory tests, take the time to note changes in your energy levels, sleep patterns, digestion, and overall well-being.

Blood Type B Brain-Boosting Diet Checklist

Eat small to moderate portions of high-quality, lean, organic meat (especially goat, lamb, and mutton) several times a week for strength, energy, and digestive health. ☐

Avoid chicken. ☐

Include regular portions of richly oiled cold-water fish. ☐

Regularly eat cultured dairy foods, such as yogurt and kefir, which are beneficial for digestive health. ☐

Eliminate wheat and corn from your diet. ☐

Eat lots of BENEFICIAL fruits and vegetables. ☐

If you need a daily dose of caffeine, replace coffee with green tea. ☐

Avoid foods that are Type B red flags, especially chicken, corn, buckwheat, peanuts, soy beans, lentils, potatoes, and tomatoes. ☐

Week 1

Blood Type Diet and Supplements

- Eliminate your most harmful AVOID foods—chicken, corn, and wheat.
- Include your most important BENEFICIAL foods on a regular schedule throughout the week. For example, have lean red meat 5 times, and omega-3-rich fish 3 to 4 times, with lots of beneficial vegetables and fruit.
- Incorporate at least 1 SUPER BENEFICIAL into your daily diet. For example, have a handful of walnuts as a snack, or eat yogurt mixed with berries for lunch.
- If you're a coffee drinker, begin to wean yourself by cutting your daily consumption in half, substituting green tea.

Exercise Regimen

- Plan to exercise at least 4 days this week, for 45 minutes each day.
  2–3 days: aerobic activity
  1–2 days: yoga or T'ai Chi
- If you have an infection or are in ill health, start slowly and gradually increase your duration and intensity of activity. The important factor is consistency. Just do it—as much as you're able.
- Use your journal to detail the time, activity, and distance. Note the number of repetitions for each exercise.

■ WEEK 1 SUCCESS STRATEGY ■
The Nitric Oxide Advantage

Nitric oxide, the combination of nitrogen and oxygen, has been shown to influence many of our most basic health processes, even including the speed and ease by which we learn. In our bodies, nitric oxide functions as a "signaling molecule." For example, it can tell the body to make blood vessels relax and widen.

Areas that are known to be influenced by nitric oxide include:

1. *Learning.* Behavioral studies show that nitric oxide may play a role in learning. Drugs that interfere with the nitric oxide signaling pathway also interfere with some types of learning tasks (e.g., spatial learning) that require long-term memory formation.

2. *Blood pressure.* Nitric oxide controls blood pressure and prevents formation of blood clots by signaling the muscles that control relaxation and expansion of blood vessels. There is some evidence that the night-time urination many people find so disturbing to their sleep may be the result of nocturnal variations in blood pressure that are caused by the fluctuations in nitric oxide activity.

3. *Heart/arteries.* When arteries become clogged, they produce less nitric oxide than normal. Treatment with nitroglycerin can increase nitric oxide, widening blood vessels and increasing blood flow. Nitric oxide also interacts with blood platelets to decrease platelet aggregation, thus lowering the risk of blood clots.

4. *Immunity.* Huge quantities of nitric oxide are produced in white blood cells to kill invading bacteria and parasites. White blood cells use nitric oxide to defend the body against tumors. Scientists are investigating whether it can be used to stop the growth of tumors.

5. *Nervous system.* Nitric oxide is synthesized in neurons of the central nervous system, where it acts as a mediator with many physiological functions, including the formation of memory, coordination between neuronal activity and blood flow, and modulation of pain.

Although anyone can benefit from healthy modulation of nitric oxide metabolism, there is some evidence that those individuals who possess the gene for the blood group B antigen (Blood Types B and AB) may be more at risk for health problems associated with imbalances in nitric oxide metabolism. Nitricycle, a supplement designed to enhance nitric oxide metabolism, is available through North American Pharmacal. Visit our Web site at www.dadamo.com.

Week 2

Blood Type Diet and Supplements

- Begin to eliminate the next level of AVOID foods—seeds, beans, and legumes that have negative lectin activity.
- Eat at least 2 to 3 BENEFICIAL animal proteins every day, from the meat, seafood, and dairy lists.
- Initially, it is best to avoid foods on the list, NEUTRAL: Allowed Infrequently.
- Continue to incorporate SUPER BENEFICIAL foods into your daily diet.
- If you're a coffee drinker, continue to cut your coffee intake, replacing it with green tea.

Exercise Regimen

- Continue to exercise at least 4 days this week, for 45 minutes each day.
  2–3 days: aerobic activity
  1–2 days: yoga or T'ai Chi
- If your work is sedentary, get in the habit of taking a couple of "movement" breaks during the day. Walk around the block or up and down stairs.

• **WEEK 2 SUCCESS STRATEGY** •
Tips for Type B Seniors

- Type Bs have a tendency to suffer memory loss and decreased mental acuity as they age. Exercise your mind by doing tasks that require concentration, such as crossword puzzles.
- A daily regimen of stretching, yoga, and meditation will lower cortisol levels and increase your mental acuity.
- Be especially careful with hygiene and safe food preparation. Type Bs are particularly vulnerable to bacterial infections. If your sense of smell has declined, and you have trouble judging freshness by smell, try to have a younger friend or relative accompany you grocery shopping.
- Maintaining a circadian rhythm—important for control of cortisol levels—can be difficult for seniors. Overall, elderly people tend to have more problems with interrupted sleep and insomnia. Ask your doctor about taking supplements of vitamin B_{12} or melatonin.

Week 3

Blood Type Diet and Supplements

- When you plan your meals for week 3, choose BENEFI-CIAL foods to replace NEUTRAL foods whenever possible. For example, choose lamb over beef, or blueberries over an apple.
- Eliminate all remaining AVOID foods.
- Liberally incorporate SUPER BENEFICIAL foods into your daily diet.

Exercise Regimen

- Continue to exercise at least 4 days this week, for 45 minutes each day.
  2–3 days: aerobic activity
  1–2 days: yoga or T'ai Chi

▪ WEEK 3 SUCCESS STRATEGY ▪
Strengthen Your Memory with Visualization

Visualization can strengthen your memory. A small study published in the June 2004 *Psychology and Aging* found that visualizing an important health task, such as taking their blood pressure or testing their blood sugar, made older adults 50 percent more likely to do it the next day than those who used other memory techniques, such as verbally repeating the task in advance. Previous research has shown that the same visualization strategy can help with everyday activities, too.

Take five minutes every night to paint a mental picture of your health tasks for the next day.

This can be especially effective for Blood Type Bs with their natural ability for visualization. I've also found that Blood Type Bs have a natural ability to relieve stress through meditation or guided imagery. I've never medicated Type B individuals who have high blood pressure without first teaching them some simple visualization techniques and sending them home to try them out for a few weeks. Those that did almost never required medication.

Here is a very simple visualization exercise to help control high blood pressure. Do this visualization two to four times daily for five to eight minutes.

Find a quiet place and make yourself comfortable and relaxed. Close your eyes and let your arms and hands lie limply on your sides or in your lap. Take a few deep breaths, inhaling through your nose and exhaling through your mouth, while imagining the red blood cells of your circulatory system coursing through your arteries and veins. See them slipping and sliding along the walls, which periodically open up like Venetian blinds to allow cells to move from the inside of the arteries out and from the outside in. Imagine the walls of your arteries relaxing and bending. Now expand the image and visualize your entire body. See the blood circulating from your heart to the arteries, to the capillaries, to the veins, then back to the lungs and heart.

Week 4

Blood Type Diet and Supplements

- Continue at the week 3 level, focusing on BENEFICIAL and SUPER BENEFICIAL foods.
- Evaluate the first 4 weeks and make adjustments.

Exercise Regimen

- Continue at the week 3 level.
- Review your progress, noting in your journal improvements in strength and flexibility. Determine which exercise regimen has worked for you, including time of day, setting, and activity level.

▪ WEEK 4 SUCCESS STRATEGY ▪

Blood Type B Berry Brain Booster

Tufts University published a study involving several antioxidant-rich extracts such as spinach and blueberries. While all scored well in enhancing memory improvement, only blueberries had a significant impact on improving motor skills like balance and coordination. While previous research has indicated that antioxidants may help lower the risk of cancer and heart disease, these new findings are the first to reveal a connection between potent antioxidants like blueberries and age-related declines. How do blueberries work? The authors of the Tufts study theorize that because blueberries keep the cell membranes healthy, they allow for more effective transport of important nutrients.

Blend together:
1 cup mixed berries (blueberries, blackberries, elderberries)
1 cup yogurt or milk*
ice

*If desired, substitute Protein Blend 4 B, available through www.dadamo.com.

Blood Type
AB

BLOOD TYPE AB DIET OUTCOME: REVERSE GENETICS

"All of my grandparents died in their sixties, my father died at seventy, and my mother died at seventy-two. I've always figured my genetics were against me, especially since I began having serious health problems (diabetes, depression, muscle pain) in my forties. I started the Type AB Diet when I was sixty-one, and after two years, I feel better than I felt at forty. My diabetes is under control, I have more energy, and at my last checkup my doctor was amazed by my test results."

Self-reported outcome from the Blood Type Diet Web site
(www.dadamo.com).

Blood Type AB: The Foods

THE BLOOD TYPE AB Fight Aging Diet is specifically adapted to provide the maximum nutritional support to fight many of the conditions associated with aging. A new category, **Super Beneficial**, highlights powerful disease-fighting foods for Blood Type AB. The **Neutral** category has also been adjusted to de-emphasize foods that are less advantageous for you. Foods designated **Neutral: Allowed Infrequently** should be minimized or avoided entirely.

Your secretor status can influence your ability to fully digest and metabolize certain foods, so various adjustments in the values are made for non-secretors. If you do not know your secretor type, the odds are that you can safely use the "secretor" values, since the majority of the population (approximately 80 percent) are secretors. However, I urge you to get tested, since the variations are important for non-secretors who want to maximize the effectiveness of the Blood Type Diet.

Blood Type AB

TOP 12 BRAIN POWER SUPER FOODS

1. soy beans and soy-based products
2. richly oiled cold-water fish (salmon, sardines)
3. cultured dairy (kefir, yogurt)
4. olive oil
5. greens (collard, kale, mustard)
6. maitake mushrooms

7. broccoli
8. berries (cherry, cranberry, gooseberry, loganberry)
9. watermelon
10. garlic
11. turmeric
12. green tea

The food charts are divided into three sections. The top of the chart suggests the average portion size and quantity per week or day, according to secretor status. These recommendations do *not* apply to the category **Neutral: Allowed Infrequently**; those foods should be eaten rarely, if at all. The charts also indicate differences in frequency for some foods, based on ethnic heritage. It has been my experience that this factor has an impact upon the individual's ability to fully digest certain foods. For the purposes of blood type food choices, persons of Hispanic heritage should follow the guidelines for Caucasians, and American Native peoples should follow the guidelines for Asians.

The middle section of the chart gives the food values. The bottom section lists variants based on secretor status.

For your convenience, we have included a number of product names (Ezekiel 4:9 bread, Worcestershire sauce, etc.). However, keep in mind that commercial formulations vary among brands and regions. For example, there are several forms of Ezekiel 4:9 bread, and not all may be right for your type. Even though a product may be listed as acceptable for you, always check its ingredients. Some products contain **Avoid** ingredients for your blood type. Of course, you may choose to make your own version of commercial products, such as bread and mayonnaise, using ingredients that suit your blood type. There are hundreds of delicious recipes for every blood type available on our Web site (www.dadamo.com) and in the book *Cook Right 4 Your Type: The Practical Kitchen Companion to* Eat Right 4 Your Type.

Meat/Poultry

Blood Type AB is somewhat better adapted to animal-based proteins than Blood Type A, mainly because of the B gene's effects on the production of enzymes involved in fat transport and digestion. However, Type AB should limit meat and avoid chicken altogether, which contains a B-immunoreactive lectin. Choose only the best quality (preferably free-range) chemical-, antibiotic-, and pesticide-free low-fat meats and poultry.

BLOOD TYPE AB: MEAT/POULTRY
Portion: 4–6 oz (men); 2–5 oz (women and children)

	African	Caucasian	Asian
Secretor	2–5	1–5	1–5
Non-Secretor	3–5	2–5	2–5
		Times per week	

SUPER BENEFICIAL	BENEFICIAL	NEUTRAL: Allowed Frequently	NEUTRAL: Allowed Infrequently	AVOID
	Lamb Mutton Rabbit	Goat Ostrich Pheasant	Liver (calf)	

SUPER BENEFICIAL	BENEFICIAL	NEUTRAL: Allowed Frequently	NEUTRAL: Allowed Infrequently	AVOID
	Turkey			All commercially processed meats
				Bacon/ham/pork
				Beef
				Buffalo
				Chicken
				Cornish hen
				Duck
				Goose
				Grouse
				Guinea hen
				Heart (beef)
				Partridge
				Quail
				Squab
				Squirrel
				Sweetbreads
				Turtle
				Veal
				Venison

Special Variants: NEUTRAL (Allowed Frequently): quail, venison.

Fish/Seafood

Richly oiled cold-water fish, such as mackerel, cod, salmon, and sardines, are especially good protein sources for Type AB, since they are excellent sources of omega-3 fatty acids and the essential fatty acids EPA and DHA, which provide fuel for brain metabolism and help control inflammation. Salmon and sardines are good sources of phosphorus, needed for energy production. Fish and seafood provide an excellent means of optimizing immune activity, which is especially important for Type AB. In general, many of the seafoods Blood Type AB must avoid have lectins with either A or B specificity, or polyamines commonly found in the foods. Avoid consuming flash-frozen fish, which has high polyamine content.

BLOOD TYPE AB: FISH/SEAFOOD
Portion: 4–6 oz (men); 2–5 oz (women and children)

	African	Caucasian	Asian
Secretor	4–6	3–5	3–5
Non-Secretor	4–7	4–6	4–6
		Times per week	

SUPER BENEFICIAL	BENEFICIAL	NEUTRAL: Allowed Frequently	NEUTRAL: Allowed Infrequently	AVOID
Cod	Grouper	Abalone	Caviar	Anchovy
Mackerel	Mahimahi	Bluefish	(sturgeon)	Barracuda

SUPER BENEFICIAL	BENEFICIAL	NEUTRAL: Allowed Frequently	NEUTRAL: Allowed Infrequently	AVOID
Salmon	Monkfish	Bullhead	Mussel	Bass (all)
Sardine	Pickerel	Butterfish	Scallops	Beluga
Sturgeon	Pike	Carp	Squid	Clam
	Porgy	Catfish	(calamari)	Conch
	Red	Chub	Whitefish	Crab
	snapper	Croaker		Eel
	Sailfish	Cusk		Flounder
	Shad	Drum		Frog
	Snail (*Helix*	Halfmoon		Gray sole
	pomatia/	fish		Haddock
	escargot)	Harvest fish		Hake
	Tuna	Herring		Halibut
		(fresh)		Herring
		Mullet		(pickled/
		Muskellunge		smoked)
		Opaleye		Lobster
		Orange		Octopus
		roughy		Oysters
		Parrot fish		Salmon
		Perch (all)		(smoked)
		Pollock		Salmon roe
		Pompano		Shrimp
		Rosefish		Sole
		Scrod		Trout (all)
		Scup		Whiting
		Shark		Yellowtail
		Smelt		

SUPER BENEFICIAL	BENEFICIAL	NEUTRAL: Allowed Frequently	NEUTRAL: Allowed Infrequently	AVOID
		Sucker		
		Sunfish		
		Swordfish		
		Tilapia		
		Tilefish		
		Tuna		
		Weakfish		

Special Variants: *Non-Secretor:* BENEFICIAL: herring (fresh); NEUTRAL (Allowed Frequently): trout (all).

Dairy/Eggs

Dairy products can be used with discretion by many Blood Type AB individuals, especially secretors. Cultured dairy foods, such as yogurt and kefir, are particularly BENEFICIAL. Kefir has been studied for its role in improving the oxygen supply to the brain. Ghee (clarified butter) is an antioxidant rich in omega-3 oils and short-chain fatty acids. Eggs, which, like fish, are a good source of docosohexaenoic acid (DHA), can complement the protein profile for your blood type. They are also an excellent source of choline, which increases energy and enhances memory. Do your best to find eggs and dairy products that are both hormone-free and organic.

BLOOD TYPE AB: EGGS
Portion: 1 egg

	African	Caucasian	Asian
Secretor	2–5	3–4	3–4
Non-Secretor	3–6	3–6	3–6
	Times per week		

BLOOD TYPE AB: MILK AND YOGURT
Portion: 4–6 oz (men); 2–5 oz (women and children)

	African	Caucasian	Asian
Secretor	2–6	3–6	1–6
Non-Secretor	0–3	0–4	0–3
	Times per week		

BLOOD TYPE AB: CHEESE
Portion: 3 oz (men); 2 oz (women and children)

	African	Caucasian	Asian
Secretor	2–3	3–4	3–4
Non-Secretor	0	0–1	0
	Times per week		

SUPER BENEFICIAL	BENEFICIAL	NEUTRAL: Allowed Frequently	NEUTRAL: Allowed Infrequently	AVOID
Ghee (clarified butter)	Cottage cheese	Casein	Cheddar	American cheese
Kefir	Egg (chicken)	Cream cheese	Colby	Blue cheese
Yogurt	Farmer cheese	Edam	Emmenthal	Brie
	Feta	Egg (goose/ quail)	Milk (cow)	Butter
	Goat cheese	Gouda	Monterey Jack	Buttermilk
	Milk (goat)	Gruyère	Sherbet	Camembert
	Mozzarella	Jarlsberg	Swiss cheese	Egg (duck)
	Ricotta	Muenster		Half-and-half
	Sour cream	Neufchâtel		Ice cream
		Paneer		Parmesan
		Quark		Provolone
		String cheese		
		Whey		

Special Variants: *Non-Secretor:* BENEFICIAL: ghee (clarified butter); NEUTRAL (Allowed Frequently): goat cheese, yogurt; AVOID: Emmenthal, Swiss cheese.

Oils

Olive oil, a monounsaturated fat, is SUPER BENEFICIAL for Blood Type AB and should be used as a primary cooking oil. Constituents in olive oil, such as flavonoids, squalenes, and polyphenols, act as powerful antioxidants. Flax (linseed) oil is high in alpha-linolenic acid, which aids brain cell connectivity.

Corn, sesame, and safflower oils can contain immunore-active proteins that impair Blood Type AB digestion. These oils can interfere with proper immune function.

BLOOD TYPE AB: OILS Portion: 1 tblsp			
	African	Caucasian	Asian
Secretor	4–7	5–8	5–7
Non-Secretor	3–6	3–6	3–4
		Times per week	

SUPER BENEFICIAL	BENEFICIAL	NEUTRAL: Allowed Frequently	NEUTRAL: Allowed Infrequently	AVOID
Flax (linseed) Olive	Walnut	Almond Black currant seed Borage seed Canola Castor Cod liver Evening primrose Peanut Soy	Wheat germ	Avocado Coconut Corn Cottonseed Safflower Sesame Sunflower

Special Variants: None.

Nuts/Seeds

Nuts and seeds can be an important secondary source of protein for Blood Type AB. Laboratory research has identified at least five natural phytochemicals in nuts that regulate the immune system and act as antioxidants. SUPER BENEFICIAL for Blood Type AB are raw flaxseeds and walnuts, which are high in omega-3 fatty acids.

BLOOD TYPE AB: NUTS/SEEDS
Portion: Whole (handful); Nut Butters (2 tblsp)

	African	Caucasian	Asian
Secretor	5–10	5–10	5–9
Non-Secretor	4–8	4–9	5–9
	Times per week		

SUPER BENEFICIAL	BENEFICIAL	NEUTRAL: Allowed Frequently	NEUTRAL: Allowed Infrequently	AVOID
Flax (linseed)	Chestnut	Almond	Brazil nut	Filbert (hazelnut)
Walnut (black/ English)	Peanut	Almond butter	Cashew	Poppy seed
	Peanut butter	Almond cheese	Cashew butter	Pumpkin seed
		Almond milk	Macadamia	Sesame butter (tahini)
		Beechnut	Pecan	
		Butternut	Pecan butter	
		Hickory	Pistachio	

SUPER BENEFICIAL	BENEFICIAL	NEUTRAL: Allowed Frequently	NEUTRAL: Allowed Infrequently	AVOID
		Lychee Pignolia (pine nut)	Safflower seed	Sesame seed Sunflower butter Sunflower seed

Special Variants: *Non-Secretor:* NEUTRAL (Allowed Frequently): peanut, peanut butter; AVOID: Brazil nut, cashew, cashew butter, pistachio.

Beans and Legumes

Blood Type AB can benefit from the vegetable proteins found in many beans and legumes. In particular, soy provides both cardiovascular and immune system benefits. Soy contains phospholipids, which help maintain brain cell membranes.

BLOOD TYPE AB: BEANS AND LEGUMES Portion: 1 cup (cooked)			
	African	Caucasian	Asian
Secretor	3–6	3–6	4–6
Non-Secretor	2–5	2–5	3–6
		Times per week	

SUPER BENEFICIAL	BENEFICIAL	NEUTRAL: Allowed Frequently	NEUTRAL: Allowed Infrequently	AVOID
Soy bean	Lentil	Bean (green/	Jicama bean	Adzuki bean
Soy cheese	(green)	snap/		Black bean
Soy milk	Navy bean	string)		Black-eyed
Soy, miso	Pinto bean	Cannellini		pea
Soy,		bean		Fava (broad)
tempeh		Copper bean		bean
Soy, tofu		Lentil		Garbanzo
		(domestic/		(chickpea)
		red)		Kidney bean
		Northern		Lima bean
		bean		Mung bean/
		Pea (green/		sprouts
		pod/snow)		
		Tamarind		
		bean		
		White bean		

Special Variants: *Non-Secretor:* NEUTRAL (Allowed Frequently): fava (broad) bean, navy bean, soy bean, soy (miso), soy (tempeh), soy (tofu); AVOID; jicama bean, soy cheese, soy milk.

Grains and Starches

Blood Type AB benefits from a moderate consumption of the proper grains for its blood type. Essene bread (manna) is SUPER BENEFICIAL. It is a 100 percent sprouted bread, from which the lectin-containing seed coat has been removed. Blood Type AB individuals—especially non-secretors—should use Essene instead of other wheat breads. Blood Type AB is also sensitive to the lectin in corn and should avoid all corn flour products.

BLOOD TYPE AB: GRAINS AND STARCHES

Portion: ½ cup dry (grains and pastas); 1 muffin; 2 slices of bread

	African	Caucasian	Asian
Secretor	6–8	6–9	6–10
Non-Secretor	4–6	5–7	6–8
		Times per week	

SUPER BENEFICIAL	BENEFICIAL	NEUTRAL: Allowed Frequently	NEUTRAL: Allowed Infrequently	AVOID
Essene bread (manna)	Amaranth	Barley	Wheat (semolina)	Buckwheat
	Ezekiel 4:9 bread	Couscous	Wheat (whole)	Cornmeal
	Millet	Quinoa	Wheat bran	Grits
	Oat bran	Spelt flour/ products	Wheat germ	Kamut
	Oat flour			Popcorn
	Oatmeal			Soba noodles (100% buckwheat)
	Rice (whole)			
	Rice (wild)			
	Rice bran			Sorghum
	Rice cake			Tapioca
	Rye (whole)			Teff

SUPER BENEFICIAL	BENEFICIAL	NEUTRAL: Allowed Frequently	NEUTRAL: Allowed Infrequently	AVOID
	Rye flour/ products Soy flour/ products Spelt (whole)			Wheat (re-fined/un-bleached) Wheat (white flour)

Special Variants: *Non-Secretor:* NEUTRAL (Allowed Frequently): Ezekiel 4:9 bread, spelt (whole); AVOID: soy flour/products, wheat (semolina), wheat (whole), wheat germ.

Vegetables

Vegetables can be your first line of defense against chronic disease. They provide a rich source of antioxidants and fiber and are essential to intestinal health. Blood Type AB SUPER BENEFICIALS include onions, which are high in quercetin, a flavonoid with potent anti-inflammatory properties, and other antioxidants that decrease oxidative stress and increase glutathione, which protects cells. Antioxidant-rich vegetables, such as broccoli, spinach, and dark greens protect against free radical damage. Broccoli is also a potent antioxidant. Mushrooms (maitake and the common domestic variety, called silver dollar) are powerful infection fighters. Cabbage—especially the juice—and cauliflower are detoxifying for Blood Type AB. Parsnips are excellent sources of vitamin C and folic acid.

An item's value also applies to its juice, unless otherwise noted.

BLOOD TYPE AB: VEGETABLES
Portion: 1 cup, prepared (cooked or raw)

	African	Caucasian	Asian
Secretor Super/ Beneficials	Unlimited	Unlimited	Unlimited
Secretor Neutrals	2–5	2–5	2–5
Non-Secretor Super/Beneficials	Unlimited	Unlimited	Unlimited
Non-Secretor Neutrals	2–3	2–3	2–3
	Times per day		

SUPER BENEFICIAL	BENEFICIAL	NEUTRAL: Allowed Frequently	NEUTRAL: Allowed Infrequently	AVOID
Broccoli	Alfalfa	Arugula	Carrot	Aloe
Cabbage	sprouts	Asparagus	Daikon	Artichoke
(juice)*	Beet	Asparagus	radish	Corn
Cauliflower	Beet greens	pea	Olive	Mushroom
Mushroom	Carrot	Bamboo	(Greek/	(abalone/
(maitake/	(juice)	shoot	green/	shiitake)
silver	Celery	Bok choy	Spanish)	Olive (black)
dollar)	Collards	Brussels	Poi	Peppers (all)
Onion (all)	Cucumber	sprouts	Potato	Pickles (all)

SUPER BENEFICIAL	BENEFICIAL	NEUTRAL: Allowed Frequently	NEUTRAL: Allowed Infrequently	AVOID
Parsnip	Dandelion	Cabbage	Pumpkin	Radish/
	Eggplant	Celeriac	Taro	sprouts
	Garlic	Chicory		Rhubarb
	Kale	Cucumber		
	Mustard	(juice)		
	greens	Endive		
	Potato	Escarole		
	(sweet)	Fennel		
	Yam	Fiddlehead		
		fern		
		Horseradish		
		Kohlrabi		
		Leek		
		Lettuce (all)		
		Mushroom		
		(enoki/		
		oyster/		
		portobello/		
		silver		
		dollar/		
		straw/tree		
		ear)		
		Okra		
		Oyster plant		
		Radicchio		
		Rappini		
		(broccoli		
		rabe)		

SUPER BENEFICIAL	BENEFICIAL	NEUTRAL: Allowed Frequently	NEUTRAL: Allowed Infrequently	AVOID
		Rutabaga		
		Scallion		
		Seaweed		
		Shallot		
		Spinach		
		Squash (all)		
		Swiss chard		
		Tomato		
		Turnip		
		Water chestnut		
		Watercress		
		Yucca		
		Zucchini		

Special Variants: *Non-Secretor:* BENEFICIAL: tomato; NEUTRAL (Allowed Frequently): beet; AVOID: poi, taro.

* To obtain the benefits of cabbage juice, it must be consumed within one minute of juicing.

Fruits and Fruit Juices

SUPER BENEFICIAL fruits for Blood Type AB include cherries, which contain pigments that inhibit intestinal toxins, and cranberries, which can help fight urinary tract infections. Other SUPER BENEFICIAL fruits have powerful antioxidant effects, particularly gooseberries and loganberries. Watermelon improves nitric oxide synthesis and reduces edema. Plums contain phytonutrients that reduce free radical damage. Blueberries have been studied for their anti-aging and antioxidant properties.

An item's value also applies to its juice, unless otherwise noted.

BLOOD TYPE AB: FRUITS AND FRUIT JUICES Portion: 1 cup			
	African	Caucasian	Asian
Secretor	3–4	3–6	3–5
Non-Secretor	1–3	2–3	3–4
			Times per day

SUPER BENEFICIAL	BENEFICIAL	NEUTRAL: Allowed Frequently	NEUTRAL: Allowed Infrequently	AVOID
Blueberry	Fig (fresh/	Apple	Apricot	Avocado
Cherry	dried)	Blackberry	Asian pear	Banana
Cranberry	Grape (all)	Boysenberry	Breadfruit	Bitter melon
Gooseberry	Grapefruit	Elderberry	Canang	Coconut
Loganberry	Kiwi	(dark blue/	melon	Dewberry
Pineapple	Lemon	purple)	Cantaloupe	Guava
Plum		Grapefruit	Casaba	Mango
Watermelon		(juice)	melon	Orange
		Kumquat	Christmas	Persimmon
		Lime	melon	Pome-
		Mulberry	Crenshaw	granate
		Muskmelon	melon	Prickly pear
		Nectarine	Currant	Quince

SUPER BENEFICIAL	BENEFICIAL	NEUTRAL: Allowed Frequently	NEUTRAL: Allowed Infrequently	AVOID
		Papaya	Date	Sago palm
		Peach	Honeydew	Star fruit
		Pear	Prune	(caram-
		Persian	Raisin	bola)
		melon	Tangerine	
		Pineapple		
		(juice)		
		Plantain		
		Raspberry		
		Spanish		
		melon		
		Strawberry		
		Youngberry		

Special Variants: *Non-Secretor:* BENEFICIAL: blackberry, blueberry, elderberry, lime; NEUTRAL (Allowed Frequently): banana; AVOID: cantaloupe, honeydew, prune, tangerine.

Spices/Condiments/Sweeteners

Many spices have medicinal properties. Garlic is a potent antioxidant. Turmeric activates an enzyme that prevents oxidation in the brain. Ginger contains an antioxidant called zingerone, which appears to have brain-protective properties.

Many common food additives, such as guar gum and carrageenan, enhance the effects of lectins found in other foods and should be avoided.

SUPER BENEFICIAL	BENEFICIAL	NEUTRAL: Allowed Frequently	NEUTRAL: Allowed Infrequently	AVOID
Cilantro (coriander leaf)	Coriander	Basil	Agar	Allspice
Garlic	Horse-radish	Bay leaf	Apple pectin	Almond extract
Ginger	Molasses (blackstrap)	Bergamot	Arrowroot	Anise
Turmeric	Oregano	Caraway	Chocolate	Aspartame
	Parsley	Cardamom	Honey	Barley malt
		Carob	Maple syrup	Carrageenan
		Chervil	Mayonnaise	Cornstarch
		Chili powder	Molasses	Corn syrup
		Chive	Rice syrup	Dextrose
		Cinnamon	Senna	Fructose
		Clove	Soy sauce	Gelatin (except veg-sourced)
		Cream of tartar	Sugar (brown/white)	Guarana
		Cumin		Gums (acacia/Arabic/guar)
		Dill		Ketchup
		Juniper		Malto-dextrin
		Licorice root*		MSG
		Mace		Pepper (black/white)
		Marjoram		
		Mint (all)		
		Mustard (dry)		
		Nutmeg		
		Paprika		
		Rosemary		
		Saffron		
		Sage		

SUPER BENEFICIAL	BENEFICIAL	NEUTRAL: Allowed Frequently	NEUTRAL: Allowed Infrequently	AVOID
		Savory		Pepper (cayenne)
		Sea salt		Pepper (peppercorn/ red flakes)
		Seaweed		
		Stevia		
		Tamari (wheat-free)		Pickle (all)
				Sucanat
		Tamarind		Tapioca
		Tarragon		Vinegar (all)
		Thyme		Worcester- shire sauce
		Vanilla		
		Wintergreen		
		Yeast (baker's/ brewer's)		

Special Variants: *Non-Secretor:* BENEFICIAL: bay leaf, yeast (brewer's); AVOID: agar, honey, juniper, maple syrup, rice syrup, sugar (brown/white).

* Do not use if you have high blood pressure.

Herbal Teas

Several herbal teas can be SUPER BENEFICIAL for Blood Type AB. Ginger contains pungent phenolic substances with pronounced antioxidative and anti-inflammatory activities. Echinacea is mildly stimulative to the immune system. Licorice root provides antiviral support and enhances cortisol modulation.

SUPER BENEFICIAL	BENEFICIAL	NEUTRAL: Allowed Frequently	NEUTRAL: Allowed Infrequently	AVOID
Echinacea	Alfalfa	Catnip	Senna	Aloe
Ginger	Burdock	Chickweed		Coltsfoot
Licorice root*	Chamomile	Dong quai		Corn silk
	Dandelion	Elder		Fenugreek
	Ginseng	Goldenseal		Gentian
	Hawthorn	Horehound		Hops
	Parsley	Mulberry		Linden
	Rosehip	Peppermint		Mullein
	Strawberry leaf	Raspberry leaf		Red clover
		Sage		Rhubarb
		Sarsaparilla		Shepherd's purse
		Slippery elm		Skullcap
		Spearmint		
		St. John's wort		
		Thyme		
		Valerian		
		Vervain		
		White birch		
		White oak bark		
		Yarrow		
		Yellow dock		

Special Variants: None.

*Do not use if you have high blood pressure.

Miscellaneous Beverages

Green tea is a SUPER BENEFICIAL beverage for Blood Type AB, because of its antioxidant and cardiovascular properties. Red wine contains gallic acid, trans-resveratrol, quercetin, and rutin—four phenolic compounds with potent antioxidant effects. Coffee should be avoided by Type AB as it exacerbates allergies.

SUPER BENEFICIAL	BENEFICIAL	NEUTRAL: Allowed Frequently	NEUTRAL: Allowed Infrequently	AVOID
Tea (green)	Wine (red)	Seltzer Soda (club) Wine (white)	Beer	Coffee (reg/ decaf) Liquor Soda (cola/ diet/ misc.) Tea, black (reg/decaf)

Special Variants: *Non-Secretor:* AVOID: beer.

Supplements

THE BLOOD TYPE AB DIET offers abundant quantities of important nutrients, such as protein and iron. However, properly calibrated supplements can provide important benefits, and this may be especially true as we age. Recent clinical studies showed that dietary supplements can treat nutritional deficiencies in the elderly, boost their immune systems, combat short-term memory loss, reduce the risk of Alzheimer's, and improve seniors' overall health. The following supplement protocols are designed for Blood Type AB individuals, to improve brain health, cognitive function, and cellular integrity.

Blood Type AB: Basic Anti-Aging Protocol

Use this protocol for 4–8 weeks, then discontinue for 2 weeks and restart.

SUPPLEMENT	ACTION	DOSAGE
High-potency vitamin-mineral complex (preferably blood type–specific)	Nutritional support	As directed
Creatine monohydrate	Increases intracellular energy and improves mental function	700 mg, 1 capsule daily
N-acetyl cysteine (NAC)	A potent antioxidant, chelating agent, and the precursor of one of the body's primary protective agents, glutathione	100 mg, 1 capsule, twice daily
Milk thistle (Silymarin)	Not only prevents the depletion of glutathione induced by alcohol and other	1–2 capsules, standardized extract, twice daily: Try to take

SUPPLEMENT	ACTION	DOSAGE
	toxic chemicals, but has been shown to increase the level of glutathione	milk thistle with a meal containing eggs, as studies have shown that when milk thistle is combined with phosphatidyl choline (found in eggs) its absorption is significantly higher

Blood Type AB:
Cognitive Improvement Protocol

Use this protocol for 4–8 weeks, then discontinue for 2 weeks and restart.

SUPPLEMENT	ACTION	DOSAGE
Brahmi (*Bacopa monnieri*)	Helps improve memory	200 mg, 1–2 capsules, twice daily
Siberian ginseng (*Eleutherococcus senticosus*)	Increases resistance to stress and aids in recovery, thus reducing adrenal and thymic atrophy	250 mg, 1 capsule, twice daily, with meals

SUPPLEMENT	ACTION	DOSAGE
OPCs (oligomeric proanthocyanidins)	Promote intestinal health	100 mg, 1 capsule daily

Blood Type AB: Immune System Health Protocol

Use this protocol for 4–8 weeks, then discontinue for 2 weeks and restart.

SUPPLEMENT	ACTION	DOSAGE
Vitamin C (from acerola cherry or rosehips)	Acts as an anti-oxidant	250 mg, 1 capsule, twice daily
Selenium	Mineral cofactor in the manufacture of glutathione peroxidase	50–100 mcg daily
Carob (*Ceratonia siliqua*)	Useful for nervous exhaustion	Solid extract, ¼–½ teaspoon, twice daily
Probiotic (preferably blood type-specific)	Promotes intestinal health	1–2 capsules, twice daily
Larch arabinogalactan	Promotes digestive and intestinal health	1 tablespoon, daily, in juice or water

Blood Type AB: Cellular Health Protocol

Use this protocol for 4–8 weeks, then discontinue for 2 weeks and restart.

SUPPLEMENT	ACTION	DOSAGE
L-arginine	Facilitates immune function and increases nitric oxide synthesis	250 mg, 1–2 capsules, twice daily
Licorice (*Glycyrrhiza sp*)*	Supports liver function; contains glycyrrhizin, which is absorbed as glycyrrhetinic acid; glycyrrhizin inhibits an enzyme called 11–beta-hydroxysteroid dehydrogenase, which converts cortisol to cortisone	1 cup of tea, twice daily, or herbal preparations under direction of a physician
Potassium citrate	Necessary for proper protein and twice daily carbohydrate metabolism; has synergies with licorice	99 mg, 1 capsule, twice daily

*Licorice can cause sodium and water retention. It should be used with a potassium supplement or in conjunction with a high-potassium diet.

The Exercise Component

FOR BLOOD TYPE AB, overall fitness is achieved with a balance of moderate aerobic activity and mentally soothing, stress-reducing exercises. Below is a list of exercises that are recommended for Blood Type AB.

EXERCISE	DURATION	FREQUENCY
Martial arts	30–60 minutes	2–3 x week
Cycling	45–60 minutes	2–3 x week
Hiking	30–60 minutes	2–3 x week
Golf (no cart!)	60–90 minutes	2–3 x week
Walking	40–50 minutes	2–3 x week
Pilates	40–50 minutes	2–3 x week
Swimming	45 minutes	2–3 x week
Yoga	40–50 minutes	1–2 x week
T'ai Chi	40–50 minutes	1–2 x week

3 Steps to Effective Exercise

1. Warm up with stretching and flexibility moves before you start your aerobic exercise.

2. To achieve maximum cardiovascular benefits, work toward an elevated heart rate that is about 70 percent of your capacity. Once you reach the elevated rate, continue exercising to maintain that rate for twenty to

thirty minutes. To calculate your maximum heart rate
and performance level:
* Subtract your age from 220.
* Multiply the difference by .70 (or .60 if you are over
age sixty). This is the high end of your performance.
* Multiply the remainder by .50. This is the low end of
  your performance.

3. Finish each aerobic session with at least a five-minute
   cooldown of stretching and relaxation moves.

Getting Started: The First Month

IF YOU ARE NEW to the Blood Type Diet, the following
guidelines will introduce you to the Blood Type AB regimen over a period of one month. Follow these recommendations as closely as possible, using a notebook to record
your personal experiences with the diet. In addition to factors that are measurable in laboratory tests, take the time to
note changes in your energy levels, sleep patterns, digestion, and overall well-being.

Blood Type AB Brain-Boosting Diet Checklist

Derive your protein primarily from sources other than
red meat. ☐

Eliminate chicken from your diet. ☐

Eat soy foods and seafood as your primary protein. ☐

Include modest amounts of cultured dairy foods in your
diet, but limit fresh milk products. ☐

Don't overdo the grains, especially wheat-derived foods.
Avoid corn flour altogether. ☐

Eat lots of BENEFICIAL fruits and vegetables, especially
those high in antioxidants and fiber. ☐

Avoid coffee, but drink two to three cups of green tea
every day. ☐

.Week 1

Blood Type Diet and Supplements

- Eliminate your most harmful AVOID foods—chicken,
  corn, buckwheat, most shellfish, and lectin-activated
  beans.
- Include your most important BENEFICIAL foods frequently throughout the week. For example, have soy-
  based foods 5 times, and omega-3-rich fish 3 to 4 times,
  with lots of BENEFICIAL vegetables and fruit.
- Incorporate at least 1 SUPER BENEFICIAL into your daily
  diet. For example, eat slices of fresh pineapple over yogurt, or sprinkle walnuts on a salad.

• If you're a coffee drinker, begin to wean yourself by cutting your daily consumption in half. Substitute green tea.

Exercise Regimen

• Plan to exercise at least 4 days this week, for 45 minutes each day.
  2 days: walking or light aerobic activity
  2 days: yoga or T'ai Chi
• Use your journal to detail the time, activity, and distance. Note the number of repetitions for each exercise.

▪ WEEK 1 SUCCESS STRATEGY ▪
The Nitric Oxide Advantage

Nitric oxide, the combination of nitrogen and oxygen, has been shown to influence many of our most basic health processes, even including the speed and ease by which we learn. In our bodies nitric oxide functions as a "signaling molecule." For example, it can tell the body to make blood vessels relax and widen.

Areas that are known to be influenced by nitric oxide include:

1. *Learning.* Behavioral studies show that nitric oxide may play a role in learning. Drugs that interfere with the nitric oxide signaling pathway also interfere with some types of learning tasks (e.g., spatial learning) that require long-term memory formation.

2. *Blood pressure.* Nitric oxide controls blood pressure and prevents formation of blood clots by signaling the muscles that control relaxation and expansion of blood vessels. There is some evi-

dence that the night-time urination many people find so disturbing to their sleep may be the result of nocturnal variations in blood pressure that are caused by the fluctuations in nitric oxide activity.

3. *Heart/arteries.* When arteries become clogged, they produce less nitric oxide than normal. Treatment with nitroglycerin can increase nitric oxide, widening blood vessels and increasing blood flow. Nitric oxide also interacts with blood platelets to decrease platelet aggregation, thus lowering the risk of blood clots.

4. *Immunity.* Huge quantities of nitric oxide are produced in white blood cells to kill invading bacteria and parasites. White blood cells use nitric oxide to defend the body against tumors. Scientists are investigating whether it can be used to stop the growth of tumors.

5. *Nervous system.* Nitric oxide is synthesized in neurons of the central nervous system, where it acts as a mediator with many physiological functions, including the formation of memory, coordination between neuronal activity and blood flow, and modulation of pain.

Although anyone can benefit from healthy modulation of nitric oxide metabolism, there is some evidence that those individuals who possess the gene for the blood group B antigen (Blood Types B and AB) may be more at risk for health problems associated with imbalances in nitric oxide metabolism. Nitricycle, a supplement designed to enhance nitric oxide metabolism, is available through North American Pharmacal. Visit our Web site at www.dadamo.com.

Week 2

Blood Type Diet and Supplements

- Begin to eliminate the next level of AVOID foods—grains, vegetables, and fruits that react poorly with Type AB blood.
- Eat 2 to 3 BENEFICIAL proteins every day.
- Continue to incorporate SUPER BENEFICIAL foods into your daily diet.
- Choose the NEUTRAL foods listed as "Allowed Frequently" over those listed "Allowed Infrequently."
- If you're a coffee drinker, continue to cut your coffee intake, replacing it with green tea.
- Manage your mealtimes to aid proper digestion. Avoid eating on the run. Make your meals relaxing, sit-down affairs. Eat slowly and chew thoroughly to encourage digestive secretions.

Exercise Regimen

- Continue to exercise at least 4 days this week, for 45 minutes each day.
  2 days: walking or light aerobic activity
  2 days: yoga or T'ai Chi
- If your work is sedentary, get in the habit of taking a couple of "movement" breaks during the day. Walk around the block or up and down stairs.

■ WEEK 2 SUCCESS STRATEGY ■
Blood Type AB Berry Brain Booster

Tufts University published a study involving several antioxidant-rich extracts such as spinach and blueberries. While all scored well in enhancing memory improvement, only blueberries had a significant impact on improving motor skills like balance and coordination. While previous research has indicated that antioxidants may help lower the risk of cancer and heart disease, these new findings are the first to reveal a connection between potent antioxidants like blueberries and age-related declines. How do blueberries work? The authors of the Tufts study theorize that because blueberries keep the cell membranes healthy, they allow for more effective transport of important nutrients.

Blend together:
1 cup mixed cranberries and blueberries
1 cup yogurt or milk*
ice

*If desired, substitute Protein Blend 4 AB, available through www.dadamo.com.

Week 3

Blood Type Diet and Supplements

- When you plan your meals for week 3, choose BENEFICIAL foods to replace NEUTRAL foods whenever possible.
- Eliminate all remaining AVOID foods.
- Liberally incorporate SUPER BENEFICIAL foods into your daily diet.
- Completely wean yourself from coffee, substituting green tea.

Exercise Regimen

- Continue to exercise at least 4 days this week, for 45 minutes each day.
  2 days: walking or light aerobic activity
  2 days: yoga or T'ai Chi

■ WEEK 3 SUCCESS STRATEGY ■
The AB Health Cocktail

Flaxseed oil is so beneficial to your health, you may want to drink this specially formulated "Membrane Fluidizer Cocktail" every day.

1 tablespoon flaxseed oil
1 tablespoon high-quality lecithin granules
6–8 ounces fruit juice

Shake well and drink.

Week 4

Blood Type Diet

- Continue at the week 3 level, focusing on BENEFICIAL and SUPER BENEFI-CIAL foods.

Exercise Regimen

- Continue at the week 3 level.
- Review your progress, noting in your journal improvements in strength and flexibility. Determine which exercise regimen has worked for you, including time of day, setting, and activity level.

■ WEEK 4 SUCCESS STRATEGY ■
Maximize Energy with the Right Eating Schedule

For Blood Type AB, the timing of your meals can be almost as important as what you eat. This is particularly true if you're trying to lose weight. The following are helpful guidelines:

- Never skip meals. You won't be "saving" calories, as the metabolic reaction will foil your efforts.
- Make breakfast your most important protein-rich meal of the day. The result will be an efficient metabolism all day long.
- Eat on a sliding scale: big breakfast, medium lunch, small dinner.
- Resist the late-night munchies, but if you have problems regulating blood sugar, have a small protein snack—yogurt or soy milk—before bedtime.

Appendices

A Simple
Definition
of Terms

agglutination: Clumping, or "gluing" together. Agglutination is one means by which the immune system defends against foreign matter and toxins, notably against lectins and opposing blood type material.

Alzheimer's disease: Amyloid plaques form in the brain, interfering with normal function. Formerly referred to as senile dementia, Alzheimer's is a progressive degenerative disease with no current cure.

antibody: The product of the immune system when it is stimulated by specific antigens. There are many classes of antibodies, among them "agglutinins," which isolate foreign substances by clumping them together so that they may be eliminated. Blood Types O, A, and B manufacture antibodies to other blood types. Blood Type AB, the universal recipient, manufactures no antibodies to other blood types.

antigen: A chemical that provokes an immune system antibody response. The blood type "ID" present on the blood cells, identified as type A or B, is one example. A type AB cell has both of these antigens. The blood type having no antigen is described as O—or "Zero." As we age, it is to our advantage to shore up our store of circulating anti–blood type antigens, as lower levels mean increased susceptibility to diseases arising from substances and organisms bearing opposing antigens.

antioxidant: Antioxidants are important, naturally occurring nutrients that help maintain health by slowing the destructive aging process of cellular molecules such as free radicals. As cells function normally in the body, they produce damaged molecules—called free radicals. Antioxidants help prevent widespread cellular destruction by willingly donating components to stabilize free radicals. Many healthy foods are rich sources of antioxidants, including the element selenium and the vitamins C, E, and A. Vitamins C and E and many plants and plant-derived substances such as green tea, quercetin, larch arabinogalactan, and milk thistle are potent antioxidants.

autoimmune diseases: Diseases generated when the cells that normally defend the body against infections mistakenly attack the body's cells, tissues, and organs.

blood type: The term commonly used to refer to the ABO blood group system. Originally used primarily to determine suitable blood and organ donor–recipient matches, ABO type determines many of the digestive and immunological characteristics of the body, as well as susceptibility to the diseases arising from infection, immune suppression, and digestive impairment. It is also one of the tools used by anthropologists to establish the origins, socioeconomic development, and movements of ancient peoples.

catecholamines: Adrenaline and noradrenaline, hormones released from the adrenal glands in response to stress.

cognitive impairment: Any dysfunction of the brain caused by traumatic brain injury, stroke, transient ischemic attacks, or the onset of senile dementia, now commonly referred to as Alzheimer's disease. Cognitive impairment implies a severe enough insult to the brain to cause a permanent loss or inability to regain full cerebral function.

cortisol: A catabolic hormone produced by the adrenal glands in response to trauma. Cortisol breaks down muscle tissue and converts the proteins from the tissue into energy. Too much cortisol can have an exhausting and destructive influence on the central nervous system.

dementia: A demonstrated lack of control of mental and emotional function indicating a permanently impaired state of function and ability to reason. Usually referred to as senile dementia, it is now considered to be a stage of Alzheimer's disease.

dopamine: A neurochemical made deep inside the brain and projected to the frontal lobes. There is a strong association between the release of dopamine and reward or reinforcement of behavior.

glutathione: A small molecule made inside almost every cell, from its three constituent amino acids: glycine, glutamate, and cysteine. Glutathione is the major antioxidant produced by the cell, protecting it from free radicals.

H-P-A Axis: The interplay of three endocrine glands—hypothalamus, pituitary, and adrenal—involved in a normal stress response.

hyperthyroidism: The overactive thyroid, conventionally treated with long-term anti-thyroid drugs or thyroidectomy, partial removal or destruction with radioactive iodine or surgery. Thyroid diseases show a preference for Blood Type O individuals. While medical intervention is recommended in the case of hyperthyroid function, reducing the types and amount of anti–blood type lectins present in the diet, especially those found in certain grains and legumes, can be of great help in resolving these conditions.

hypothyroidism: Underproduction of thyroid hormone, thyroxine (t3) and/or free triiodothyronine (t4). Conventionally treated by hormone replacement therapy. Thyroid conditions often respond favorably to a blood type–appropriate diet.

immune system: The physiological determination of and response to "self" and "non-self" accomplished through the action of many organs and cells throughout the body, essential to the preservation of its health and integrity.

lectins: Proteins that attach to preferred receptors in the human body. Food lectins are often blood type–specific. A lectin's action may initiate agglutination, inflammation, the abnormal proliferation of cells of the immune and nervous systems, or insulin resistance, depending upon the type of cells targeted. Abundant in the vegetable kingdom, lectins are fewer in number and type among animal foods.

metabolism: The aggregate of physical and chemical processes by which organisms maintain life, in the opposing functions of building tissue (anabolism) and breaking down tissue and foreign matter to be used as fuel (catabolism).

mitochondria: Energy-producing particles in the cells.

nitric oxide: A short-lived molecule crucial to the regulation of the central nervous system.

polyamines: A group of cell components (putrescine, spermidine, and spermine) that are important in the regulation of cell proliferation and cell differentiation. There is also evidence suggesting a role for polyamines in programmed cell death. Although their exact functions have not yet been identified, it is clear that polyamines play important roles in a number of cellular processes.

selectins: Proteins that mediate the binding of white blood cells to the walls of the blood vessels, signaling the initiation of the inflammatory response.

stroke: A brain attack as opposed to a heart attack, stroke is considered the third leading cause of death in the United States. Usually, an ischemic stroke is caused by a blood clot blocking the flow of blood through the brain. If there is bleeding into and around the brain, it is referred to as a hemorrhagic stroke, or a cerebro-vascular accident. Smaller strokes are referred to as transient ischemic attacks. Many strokes are fatal. If promptly and properly treated, some strokes and their effects are reversible. A clot-busting drug called TPA is sometimes administered.

transient ischemic attacks: Small, or petit, strokes. Some people may suffer from a bombardment of these "minor" strokes, slowly losing function over time. Others seem to shrug them off and continue to perform relatively well, depending upon which part of the brain is affected.

traumatic brain injury: More than 5 million Americans are living with traumatic brain injuries. Some are severely impaired, others less so, but all are suffering from the effects of a trauma to the brain. Most of these traumatic injuries occur as the result of vehicular accidents, some as the result of sports injuries, some because of accidental falls. Mental acuity, emotional stability, verbal and speech skills, and physical abilities all may be affected.

FAQs:
The Blood
Type Diet®

Susceptibility to various diseases according to blood type (such as the high rate of cancer in Blood Type A) has been studied in people who didn't necessarily eat right for their blood type. How much do you project that these statistics will change for people who *do* eat right for their type?

Let's take cancer as an example. It has been speculated that 35 percent of all cancers are the result of genetic outcome, 35 percent the result of diet, and 30 percent the result of environment, principally smoking. If we assume that most (say, 80 percent) of the dietary causes will be eliminated when you follow the Blood Type Diet; that you don't smoke; and that understanding blood type susceptibilities (such as stress links) allows you to circumvent about 25 percent of the genetically determined cancers, I would estimate the following benefit:

- Environmental causes reduced 5 to 8 percent from not smoking.

- Dietary causes reduced about 7 percent from the Blood Type Diet.

- Effects of blood type on other susceptibilities and genetic causes reduced about 28 to 29 percent.

The bottom line: The cancer rate is cut roughly in half for Type A individuals following the Blood Type Diet—which is what I have observed in my practice.

I take medication for an illness. Can I stop taking it if I'm on the Blood Type Diet?

Never stop taking a prescribed medication without consulting your physician. In fact, I strongly urge you to discuss the diet and supplement recommendations with your doctor before embarking on the Blood Type Diet.

An herb that is an AVOID for my blood type has been recommended by my naturopath. How should I proceed?

This will require some discernment on your part. An herb is generally considered an AVOID for a blood type due to particular negative metabolic reactions that may be induced by the herb or indirectly induced as a side effect. If possible, attempt to locate a similarly functioning herb with similar benefits.

Generally, a supplement is considered an AVOID because it is bountiful in a well-rounded, fresh food–based diet for your blood type. Additional supplementation could be considered toxic. However, if you have a diagnosed deficiency of the substance, or a medical condition shown to benefit by supplementation, then the supplement may be taken. It is always wise to consult a nutritionally knowledgeable person who can monitor your health in this situation.

What constitutes an acceptable level of compliance with the Blood Type Diet?

If you are recovering from an illness or want to lose weight, 80 to 100 percent of your food choices should be SUPER BENEFICIAL. If you are a healthy individual over the age of fifty-five, 80 percent of foods should be HIGHLY BENEFICIAL. If you are under fifty-five and healthy, 70 percent or more of your food choices should be HIGHLY BENEFICIAL. The remainder of your food choices should be NEUTRAL. AVOIDs should not be eaten.

Since tomatoes are not allowed on the Type A or B diets, what is a good source of lycopene?

First, keep in mind that tossing a tomato into your salad is not going to give you all that much lycopene. Tomatoes have a very high water content, so you only find high concentrations of lycopene in tomato paste. Unfortunately, there are also large amounts of tomato lectin in tomato paste. However, lycopene is found in a number of other foods in addition to tomatoes. Excellent sources include guava, red grapefruit, watermelon, papaya, and apricot.

One of my friends sees a naturopathic doctor who claims that naturopathic philosophy is based exclusively on vegetarian-based diets.

It is a deeply ingrained idea for some people that any consumption of animal products is automatically prohibited in a naturopathic diet. I have even had some individuals within my own profession suggest that I had abandoned the core of naturopathic medicine by advocating good-quality meat for individuals of certain blood types. It's important to ask, what does the evidence show? Naturopathic medicine developed from the water cure movement of Europe. Theodore Hahn is credited as being the first of the pioneers of this water cure movement to integrate vegetarian dietetic principles. He was convinced that a meat-free diet would prolong life. In fact he was so convinced of the value of a vegetarian diet that he spent a great deal of his professional life writing books and pamphlets on the subject and was the editor of a magazine called *The Vegetarian*. He died of colon cancer at the age of fifty-nine. The point is, one diet does not fit all, and you should be suspicious of any diet philosophy that says it can.

Should I avoid genetically engineered food?

Yes! Genetic engineering moves lectin molecules from one species to another. Since lectins are the molecules that interact with our blood types, an otherwise allowable food can easily become an AVOID. Currently, the only way to safely avoid genetically engineered foods is to choose organic.

How is alpha-lipoic acid used in the treatment of Alzheimer's disease?

Since oxidative stress and energy depletion are characteristic biochemical hallmarks of Alzheimer's disease, antioxidants with positive effects on glucose metabolism, such as alpha-lipoic acid, may exert positive effects in these patients. In one study, 600 mg of alpha-lipoic acid was given daily to nine patients with Alzheimer's disease and related dementias. The treatment led to a stabilization of cognitive functions in the study group, demonstrated by constant scores in two neuropsychological tests. Despite the fact that this study was small and not randomized, this is the first indication that treatment with alpha-lipoic acid might be a successful neuroprotective therapy for Alzheimer's disease and related dementias.

Why do you recommend the methylcobalamin form of vitamin B_{12}?

This coenzyme form of B_{12} is believed to be a much more active form of the vitamin. It appears to be better absorbed and retained in higher amounts within the tissues—particularly in the liver, brain, and nervous system.

My husband is Type O, and when he takes a licorice supplement he feels that it reduces his sexual potency. Is there a connection between licorice and sexual ability?

Large doses of licorice have been known to cause breast tenderness in men. (I remember in our school's clinic a case of a man with rather large breast enlargement due to drinking more than one gallon of strong licorice tea every day over a period of two years.) Licorice has been shown to lower testosterone and to bind with estrogen receptors. In limited amounts and in nonsensitive individuals, this is probably not much of an issue; however, people do vary significantly in their sensitivity to licorice, and prudence should be used with taking licorice or any other herbal supplement. Your husband may want to switch over to using DGL licorice, as this form still possesses many of licorice's beneficial properties while eliminating the potential for its more serious side effects, such as edema (swelling), high blood pressure, and sexual side effects.

My wife has been diagnosed with kidney failure (around 13 percent functional, according to tests), and I wanted to know if your diet program would be of any help to her condition. She does not desire a kidney transplant or dialysis.

Dietary lectins have been shown to increase antibodies against the kidney glomerulus (the filtration device used to detoxify the blood). Following the Blood Type Diet can help prevent this, since it minimizes exposure to foods that may contain problematic lectins.

Another suggestion is to use certain types of dietary fibers to help eliminate poisons that can build up in a person with compromised kidney function. Larch arabinogalactan has been studied for its ability in inhibiting colonic bacterial ammonia generation and increasing fecal nitrogen excretion. Studies showed that larch arabinogalactan decreased mean plasma urea in uremic subjects by 11 percent over a period of six to eight weeks.

I am a Type O American Indian, type 2 diabetic, with diverticulosis, which has caused severe constipation over the last six months. Can the diet help me?

Many people have small pouches in their colons that

bulge outward through weak spots, like an inner tube that pokes through weak places in a tire. Each pouch is called a diverticulum. Pouches (plural) are called diverticula. The condition of having diverticula is called diverticulosis. About half of all Americans age sixty to eighty, and almost everyone over age eighty, have diverticulosis.

In general, following the Type O Diet, with emphasis on lots of BENEFICIAL fruits and vegetables, plus lean meats, can help regulate bowel function, especially if you make it part of a program that includes regular exercise.

For some type 2 diabetics, diet and exercise are sufficient to keep the disease under control. However, you must see your doctor regularly, especially if you have any change of symptoms. Supplementing the diet with fenugreek seeds has been shown in clinical and experimental studies to reduce blood glucose and insulin levels while also lowering blood cholesterol. Adding several helpings of allowable mushrooms to the diet may also help with managing type 2 diabetes. Finally, supplementing with the antioxidant quercetin may help control diabetic complications in some individuals.

How does meditation reduce stress and improve cognitive function?

Of all meditation techniques, "TM," or transcendental meditation, is the best studied for its antistress effects. Studies have shown that catecholamines in the urine decrease during and following TM meditation.

This would be of advantage to Blood Type O, who has trouble clearing catecholamines. Even more significant, for Blood Types A and B, it appears that regular practice of TM results in lower resting basal cortisol levels for many practi-

tioners. It is quite likely that these antistress results of meditation are available from other forms of meditation as well.

Meditation and visualization appear to be especially effective for Types B and AB individuals, though it can be
practiced by all blood types. The combination of music
with guided imagery appears to be a very useful method
for lowering high cortisol.

**I thought nitric oxide was a dangerous substance, but you say
it plays many positive roles, especially for Types B and AB.**

Renewed interest in the neurotransmitter nitric oxide
has researchers looking at its precursor, L-arginine, for
treating certain kinds of heart disease. Once thought to be
only a dangerous environmental pollutant and a poison, nitric oxide is now known to be made in the body and to play
numerous roles, including brain activity regulation and circulation control.

Using nitric oxide for vasodilation, the widening of
blood vessels, has been a common practice for a long time
but has only recently been understood. During World War I,
doctors noticed that workers in ammunition factories who
were packing shells with nitroglycerin had very low blood
pressures. The observation eventually led to the development
of a nitroglycerin pill for the rapid relief of angina—that is,
exercise-induced chest pain caused by oxygen deficiency in
the heart. In 1987, nitric oxide was determined to be the re-
laxant factor released by endothelial cells, explaining how
nitroglycerin tablets help angina sufferers.

Nitric oxide controls blood pressure and prevents formation of blood clots by signaling the muscles that control
relaxation and expansion of blood vessels. There is some
evidence that the night-time urination many people find
so disturbing to their sleep may be the result of nocturnal

variations in blood pressure that are the result of the fluctuations in nitric oxide activity.

When arteries become clogged, they produce less nitric
oxide than normal. Treatment with nitroglycerin can increase nitric oxide, widening blood vessels and increasing
blood flow. Nitric oxide also interacts with blood platelets
to decrease platelet aggregation, thus lowering the risk of
blood clots.

Resources and Products

General

National Institute on Aging
7201 Wisconsin Avenue, MSC 9205
Bethesda, MD 20892-9205
www.nia.nih.gov

Centers for Disease Control and Prevention
1600 Clifton Road
Atlanta, GA 30333
404-639-1388 or 1-888-232-3228
www.cdc.gov/ncidod/diseases/cfs

Environmental Research Foundation
P.O. Box 5036
Annapolis, MD 21403
410-263-1584
www.rachel.org

The Institute for Human Individuality
Southwest College of Naturopathic Medicine
2140 E. Broadway Road
Tempe, AZ 85282
480-858-9100
www.ifhi-online.org

The Institute for Human Individuality is under the 501c3 status of Southwest College of Naturopathic Medicine. Its prime goal is to foster research in the expanding area of human nutrigenomics. Nutrigenomics seeks to provide a molecular understanding for how common dietary chemicals affect health by altering the expression or structure of an individual's genetic makeup. (IFHI is currently conducting a twelve-week randomized, double-blind, controlled trial implementing the Blood Type Diet to determine its effects on the outcomes of patients with rheumatoid arthritis.)

Blood Type–Specific Resources

Dr. Peter D'Adamo

The D'Adamo Naturopathic Center in Wilton, Connecticut, blends time-honored natural healing techniques with state-of-the-art diagnostics. The clinic staff is comprised of naturopathic physicians (N.D.s) working with medical doctors (M.D.s), nurses (R.N.s), and other licensed health professionals, all under the precepts and guidance of Dr. Peter D'Adamo. To find out more or to schedule an appointment, please contact:

The D'Adamo Naturopathic Center
213 Danbury Road
Wilton, CT 06897
203-834-7500

www.dadamo.com

The World Wide Web has proven to be a valuable venue for exploring and applying the tenets of the Blood Type Diet and lifestyle. Since January 1997, hundreds of thousands have visited the site to participate in the ABO chat groups, to peruse the scientific archives, to share experiences and recipes, and to learn more about the science of blood type.

Blood Type Specialty Products and Supplements

North American Pharmacal, Inc., is the official distributor of Blood Type specialty products. The product line includes supplements, books, tapes, teas, meal replacement bars, cosmetics, and support material that make eating and living right for your type easier.

North American Pharmacal, Inc.
213 Danbury Road
Wilton, CT 06897
Toll-free: 877-ABO TYPE (877-226-8973)
www.4yourtype.com

Home Blood-Typing Kits

North American Pharmacal, Inc., is the official distributor of Home Blood Type Testing Kits. Each kit costs $9.95 (plus shipping and handling) and is a single-use, disposable, educational device capable of determining one individual's ABO and Rhesus (Rh) blood type. Results are obtained within about four to five minutes. If you have several friends or family members who need to learn their blood type, you will need to order a separate home blood-typing kit for each individual.

The Blood Type Library

The following books are available in bookstores, health-food stores, selected grocery and specialty stores, on the Web, and through North American Pharmacal.

Eat Right 4 Your Type
The Individualized Diet Solution to Staying Healthy, Living Longer, and Achieving Your Ideal Weight
By Dr. Peter J. D'Adamo, with Catherine Whitney
G. P. Putnam's Sons, 1996

The original Blood Type Diet book, with over two million copies sold in more than sixty-five languages.

Cook Right 4 Your Type
The Practical Kitchen Companion to Eat Right 4 Your Type
By Dr. Peter J. D'Adamo, with Catherine Whitney
G. P. Putnam's Sons, 1998 (Berkley Trade Paperback, 1999)

Includes over two hundred original recipes, thirty-day meal plans, and guidelines for each blood type.

Live Right 4 Your Type
The Individualized Prescription for Maximizing Health, Metabolism, and Vitality in Every Stage of Your Life
By Dr. Peter J. D'Adamo, with Catherine Whitney
G. P. Putnam's Sons, 2001

A total health and lifestyle plan based on the individual variations observed for each blood type. Includes new research on the mind-body connection and the importance of blood type secretor status.

Eat Right 4 Your Type Complete Blood Type Encyclopedia
By Dr. Peter J. D'Adamo, with Catherine Whitney
Riverhead Books, 2002

The A-to-Z reference guide for the blood type connection to symptoms, disease, conditions, medications, vitamins, supplements, herbs, and food.

4 Your Type Pocket Guides
Blood Type, Food, Beverage, and Supplement Lists
By Peter J. D'Adamo, with Catherine Whitney
Berkley Books, 2002

The Eat Right 4 Your Type Portable and Personal Blood Type Guides are pocket-sized and user-friendly. They serve as a handy reference tool while shopping, cooking, and eating out. Each book contains the food, beverage, and supplement list for each blood type plus handy tips and ideas for incorporating the Blood Type Diet into your daily life.

Eat Right 4 Your Baby
The Individualized Guide to Fertility and Maximum Health During Pregnancy, Nursing, and Your Baby's First Year

By Dr. Peter J. D'Adamo, with Catherine Whitney
G. P. Putnam's Sons, 2003

An invaluable guide for couples looking to combine the best of naturopathic and blood type science to maximize the health of mother and baby—with practical blood type–specific guidelines for achieving a healthy state before pregnancy, eating and living right during pregnancy, and continuing in good health during baby's first year.

Dr. Peter J. D'Adamo's Eat Right 4 (for) Your Type Health Library

Allergies: Fight Them with the Blood Type Diet®
Arthritis: Fight It with the Blood Type Diet®
Cancer: Fight It with the Blood Type Diet®
Cardiovascular Disease: Fight It with the Blood Type Diet®
Diabetes: Fight It with the Blood Type Diet®
Fatigue: Fight It with the Blood Type Diet®
Menopause: Manage Its Symptoms with the Blood Type Diet®

Index

acetyl L-carnitine, 34, 69
adenosine, 49
aerobic exercise, 71–72
African Americans, 131
agglutination, 20, 22, 207
aging
  and blood type, 17–27
  of brain, 13–15
  and diet, 21–23
  four keys to fighting, 28–37
ALA (alpha-lipoic acid), 34–35,
  68, 217
alcohol, 150
allyl methyl trisulfide, 139–140
alpha-linolenic acid, 52, 91, 133,
  176
Alzheimer's disease, 13–15, 23,
  207, 217
amino acids, 94
Amla/Indian gooseberry, 69
amyloid plaques, 13
animal protein, 84
anti-aging profile, 24–26

anti-aging protocol
  for Blood Type A, 109–110
  for Blood Type AB, 192–193
  for Blood Type B, 151–152
  for Blood Type O, 68–69
antibody, 17–19, 22–23, 207
antigen, 17–19, 208
antioxidants, 14, 208
Asians, 131
ATP (adenosine triphosphate), 37
autoimmune diseases, 17–20, 208

baby boomers, 15–16
bacteria
  friendly, 33
  infections from, 162
bananas, 60, 101
beans/legumes
  for Blood Type A, 94–95
  for Blood Type AB, 179–180
  for Blood Type B, 136–137
  for Blood Type O, 55–56
betaine hydrochloride, 109

beverages. *See also* herbal teas
  for Blood Type A, 107–108
  for Blood Type AB, 191
  for Blood Type B, 150
  for Blood Type O, 66–67
biological individuality, 4–5
blackberries, 101
bladderwrack, 71
blood type, 208. *See also*
      individual blood types
  and aging, 17–27
  anti-aging profile, 24–26
  frequently asked questions,
      213–221
  and longevity, 26–27
  resources/products, 223–228
Blood Type A, 81
  anti-aging profile, 24–25
  anti-aging protocol, 109–110
  cellular health protocol,
      113–114
  cognitive improvement
      protocol, 110–111
  exercise for, 114–115
  first month regimen for,
      116–123
  foods for, 82–84
    beans/legumes, 94–95
    beverages, 107–108
    dairy/eggs, 88–91
    fish/seafood, 86–88
    fruits/fruit juices, 101–103
    grains/starches, 95–97
    herbal teas, 106–107
    meat/poultry, 84–85
    nuts/seeds, 92–94
    oils, 91–92
    spices/condiments/
      sweeteners, 103–105
    super foods, 83
    vegetables, 97–100
  immune system protocol,
      111–112
  supplements for, 108–114

Blood Type AB, 167
  anti-aging profile, 25
  anti-aging protocol, 192–193
  cellular health protocol, 195
  cognitive improvement
      protocol, 193–194
  exercise for, 196–197
  first month regimen for,
      197–204
  foods for, 168–170
    beans/legumes, 179–180
    beverages, 191
    dairy/eggs, 174–176
    fish/seafood, 172–174
    fruits/fruit juices, 185–187
    grains/starches, 180–182
    herbal teas, 189–190
    meat/poultry, 170–171
    nuts/seeds, 178–179
    oils, 176–177
    spices/condiments/
      sweeteners, 187–189
    super foods, 168–169
    vegetables, 182–185
  immune system protocol, 194
  supplements for, 191–195
Blood Type B, 124
  anti-aging profile, 25
  anti-aging protocol, 151–152
  cellular health protocol, 154
  cognitive improvement
      protocol, 152
  exercise for, 155–156
  first month regimen for,
      156–166
  foods for, 124–126
    beans/legumes, 136–137
    beverages, 150
    dairy/eggs, 131–133
    fish/seafood, 128–130
    fruits/fruit juices, 143–145
    grains/starches, 138–139
    herbal teas, 148–149
    meat/poultry, 126–128

nuts/seeds, 134–136
oils, 133–134
spices/condiments/
sweeteners, 146–148
super foods, 125
vegetables, 139–143
immune system protocol, 153
supplements for, 150–154
Blood Type O, 41–42, 218–219
anti-aging profile, 24
anti-aging protocol, 68–69
cellular health protocol, 71
cognitive improvement
protocol, 69–70
exercise for, 71–73
first month regimen for, 73–80
foods for, 42–44
beans/legumes, 55–56
beverages, 66–67
dairy/eggs, 49–53
fish/seafood, 46–48
fruits/fruit juices, 60–62
grains/starches, 56–57
herbal teas, 65–66
meat/poultry, 44–45
nuts/seeds, 53–54
oils, 52–53
spices/condiments/
sweeteners, 62–65
super foods, 43
vegetables, 58–60
immune system protocol, 70
supplements for, 67–71
blueberries, 60, 78–79, 101,
120, 143, 165–166, 186,
202
Brahmi, 110, 193
brain
aging process, 9–13
exercises for, 75–76
foods for, 28–29
injury to, 12
and lectins, 23
and soy, 30–32

super foods for, 43
supplements for, 35–36
brain-derived neurotrophic factor
(BDNF), 71–72
broccoli, 97, 139–140, 182
Brussels sprouts, 139
buttermilk, 131
butyrate, 49
B vitamins, 15, 29, 35, 68, 69, 88

cabbage, 139, 182
caffeine, 65, 107
cancer rate, 213–214
caprylic acid, 70
carob, 153, 194
carrageenan, 63, 103, 146
catecholamines, 209
Caucasians, 131
cauliflower, 139, 182
caviar, 128
cayenne pepper, 63, 146
cellular health protocol
for Blood Type A, 113–114
for Blood Type AB, 195
for Blood Type B, 154
for Blood Type O, 71
chamomile tea, 106
cheese, 131
cherries, 101, 185
Chi breathing, 118
chicken, 127, 170
chlorogenic acid, 101, 143
choline, 49, 88, 131, 174
circulatory problems, 11
cod, 172
coffee, 66–67, 107, 150, 191
cognitive impairment, 12, 209
cognitive improvement protocol
for Blood Type A, 110–111
for Blood Type AB, 193–194
for Blood Type B, 152
for Blood Type O, 69–70
cold-water fish, 46, 86, 128, 172
coleus, 71

compliance level, 215
condiments. *See* spices/
    condiments/sweeteners
conjugated linoleic acid (CLA),
    44
CoQ-10, 34
corn, 95, 138, 140, 181
corn oil, 133, 177
coronary heart disease, 91
cortisol, 12, 121, 148, 162, 189,
    209
cranberries, 143, 185
creatine monohydrate, 44, 152,
    192

dairy/eggs
    for Blood Type A, 88–91
    for Blood Type AB, 174–176
    for Blood Type B, 131–133
    for Blood Type O, 49–53
dandelions, 97–98
dandelion tea, 65, 106
dementia, 13–15, 209
denture stomatitis, 80
DHA (docosahexaenoic acid), 36,
    49, 68, 86, 88, 111, 128,
    131, 172, 174
diet
    and aging, 21–23
    for Blood Type A, 82–108
    for Blood Type AB, 168–191
    for Blood Type B, 124–150
    for Blood Type O, 42–67
digestion, 22, 29
dithiolthiones, 140
diverticulosis, 219
DMAE, 70

eating schedule, 123, 204
echinacea tea, 106, 189
eggs. *See* dairy/eggs
elderberries, 101, 143
elective surgery, 80

EPA (eicosapentaenoic acid), 49,
    86, 128, 172
escarole, 97
Essene bread, 56, 138, 181
ethnic heritage, 43, 82, 126, 169
eucommia bark, 153
exercise, 14–15, 32–33
    for Blood Type A, 114–115
    for Blood Type AB, 196–197
    for Blood Type B, 155–156
    for Blood Type O, 71–73
Ezekiel 4:9 bread, 44, 126, 169

false insulin, 23
fiber, 139, 182
first month regimen
    for Blood Type A, 116–123
    for Blood Type AB, 197–204
    for Blood Type B, 156–166
    for Blood Type O, 73–80
fish/seafood
    for Blood Type A, 86–88
    for Blood Type AB,
        172–174
    for Blood Type B, 128–130
    for Blood Type O, 46–48
flavonoids, 133
flax oil, 176
flaxseeds, 53, 91, 92, 134, 178
folate, 15
folic acid, 69, 97
foods
    for Blood Type A, 82–108
    for Blood Type AB, 168–191
    for Blood Type B, 124–150
    for Blood Type O, 42–67
free radicals, 11, 14, 58, 182
frequently asked questions,
    213–221
frozen fish, 172
fruits/fruit juices
    for Blood Type A, 101–103
    for Blood Type AB, 185–187

for Blood Type B, 143–145
for Blood Type O, 60–62
fucose, 58

galectin, 127
gallic acid, 107, 191
garlic, 62–63, 103
genetically engineered food, 216
ghee, 49, 131, 174
ginger, 63, 103, 146
ginger tea, 106, 189
ginkgo biloba, 36, 152
ginseng, 37
ginseng tea, 65, 148
glossary of terms, 207–212
glutamine, 35
glutathione, 97, 182, 209
glycosylated sugars, 23
Gokharu/Caltrop, 152
gooseberries, 185
grains/starches
    for Blood Type A, 95–97
    for Blood Type AB, 180–182
    for Blood Type B, 138–139
    for Blood Type O, 56–57
grass-fed beef, 44, 127
green drinks, 36
green leafy vegetables, 58
green tea, 36, 67, 71, 107, 114,
    191
guar gum, 63, 103, 146

halibut, 128
Harris Interactive survey, 15
hatha yoga, 114
herbal teas. *See also* beverages
    for Blood Type A, 106–107
    for Blood Type AB, 189–190
    for Blood Type B, 148–149
    for Blood Type O, 65–66
hippocampus, 13
Hispanics, 43, 82, 126, 169
holy basil tea, 106

hormonal deficiency, 11
H-P-A axis, 35, 209
hydrochloric acid, 25
hypertension, 11
hyperthyroidism, 210
hypothyroidism, 210

immune system, 18, 92, 189, 210
    life cycle, 19–20
immune system protocol
    for Blood Type A, 111–112
    for Blood Type AB, 194
    for Blood Type B, 153
    for Blood Type O, 70
inflammation, 22
insulin resistance, 23
intestinal alkaline phosphatase,
    25, 98
isoflavones, 94

kale, 97
Katz, Lawrence, Dr., 75–76
Keep Your Brain Alive (Katz and
    Rubin), 75–76
kefir, 131, 174
kidney failure, 23, 218

larch arabinogalactan, 70, 153,
    194, 218
l-arginine, 154, 195
lectins, 21–23, 63, 103, 135, 136,
    146, 170, 210, 218
legumes. *See* beans/legumes
licorice, 146, 148, 154, 189, 195,
    217–218
linolenic acid, 58
lipoic acid, 34–35
loganberries, 185
longevity, 26–27
lycopene sources, 215

magnesium citrate, 151
maitake mushroom, 58, 139, 153

malic acid, 113
meat/poultry
   for Blood Type A, 84–85
   for Blood Type AB, 170–171
   for Blood Type B, 126–128
   for Blood Type O, 44–45
medication, 214
meditation, 219–220
melatonin, 36
memory loss, 9, 13–15, 35–36, 162
metabolism, 10–13, 210
milk thistle, 111–112, 192–193
mitochondria, 10–11, 34–35, 210
mitogen, 22
mung beans, 136
mushrooms, 58, 139, 153, 182

NAC (N-acetyl cysteine), 109, 192
NADH (nicotinamide adenine dinucleotide), 37
Native Americans, 43, 82, 126, 169
naturopathy, 216
neochlorogenic acid, 101, 143
nervous system balance, 37
Neurology, 15
nitric oxide, 12, 143, 159–160, 185, 199–200, 211, 220–221
NK (Natural Killer) cells, 32
non-secretor, 21, 84, 95, 125, 131, 138, 140, 143, 168–169, 181
NSAIDs (nonsteroidal anti-inflammatory drugs), 80
nutrient deficiency, 13
Nutrition, 15
nuts/seeds
   for Blood Type A, 92–94
   for Blood Type AB, 178–179
   for Blood Type B, 134–136
   for Blood Type O, 53–54

oats, 56
oils
   for Blood Type A, 91–92
   for Blood Type AB, 176–177
   for Blood Type B, 133–134
   for Blood Type O, 52–53
okra, 97
olive oil, 52, 91, 133, 176
omega-3 fatty acids, 44, 49, 53, 86, 92, 128, 172, 174, 178
omega-6 fatty acids, 52
onions, 58, 97, 139, 182
OPCs (oligomeric proanthocyanidins), 110, 194
oranges, 101
osteoporosis, 25

pantethine, 113
pantothenic acid, 88, 131
parsnips, 97, 182
phenylalanine, 98
phosphatidylserine, 35
phospholipids, 35, 94, 179
phosphorus, 128, 172
phytochemicals, 92, 101, 143, 178, 185
pineal gland, 36
plant enzyme formula, 109
plums, 60, 101, 143, 185–186
polyamines, 172, 211
polyphenols, 133, 150
potassium citrate, 154, 195
poultry. See meat/poultry
premature aging, 10–13
probiotics, 70, 77, 110, 194
protein, 80
prunes, 101
Psychology and Aging, 163

quercetin, 58, 97, 107, 112, 182, 191

reactive plasticity, 23
red wine, 107, 150, 191
resources/products, 223–228
rosehip tea, 106
Rubin, Manning, 75–76
Russian rhodiola, 69
rutin, 107, 191

safflower oil, 177
salmon, 128, 172
sardines, 128, 172
sarsaparilla tea, 65
seafood. See fish/seafood
seaweed, 58
secretor, 21, 84, 125, 140,
     168–169
seeds. See nuts/seeds
selectins, 211
selenium, 112, 194
sesame oil, 133, 177
sesame seeds, 135
shiitake mushroom, 139
Siberian ginseng, 112, 152,
     193
sleep, 121–122
soy, 30–32, 94, 136, 179
spices/condiments/sweeteners
     for Blood Type A, 103–105
     for Blood Type AB,
          187–189
     for Blood Type B, 146–148
     for Blood Type O, 62–65
spinach, 97, 182
spreading hogweed, 111
sprouted food complex, 110
sprouted grains, 138, 180
squalenes, 133
starches. See grains/starches
strength-training, 72
stress, 12
stroke, 11, 211
sunflower oil, 133
sunflower seeds, 135
Super Beneficials, 2

super foods
     for Blood Type A, 83
     for Blood Type AB, 168–169
     for Blood Type B, 125
     for Blood Type O, 43
supplements, 15, 214–215
     antioxidants, 36
          for Blood Type A, 108–114
          for Blood Type AB, 191–195
          for Blood Type B, 150–154
          for Blood Type O, 67–71
     for brain cell activity, 35–36
     for mitochondrial function/
          repair, 34–35
     for nervous system balance,
          37
     for vascular health, 36
sweeteners. See spices/
          condiments/sweeteners
Swiss chard, 97

T'ai Chi, 114
tomatoes, 98, 140
toxins, 33–34, 77, 139, 185
transcendental meditation,
     219–220
transient ischemic attack, 211
trans resveratrol, 107, 191
traumatic brain injury, 12,
     211–212
triglycerides, 91
Tufts University, 78–79, 165, 202
tumor, 12
turkey, 127
turmeric, 62, 103, 146

vascular health, 36
vegetables
     for Blood Type A, 97–100
     for Blood Type AB, 182–185
     for Blood Type B, 139–143
     for Blood Type O, 58–60
vegetarianism, 216
vigorous exercise, 71–72

vinpocetine, 151
visualization, 163–164, 220
Vitamin A, 36
Vitamin B$_1$ (thiamine
    hydrochloride), 69
Vitamin B$_5$ (pantothenic acid), 35
Vitamin B$_{12}$ (methylcobalamin),
    15, 35, 68, 110, 122, 217
Vitamin C, 36, 97, 194
Vitamin E, 36
vitamin-mineral complex, 68,
    109, 151, 192

walking, 114, 115
walnut oil, 91
walnuts, 53, 92, 134, 178
watermelon, 143, 185
wheat, 56, 95, 138, 146
White, Lon, Dr., 30–32

yams, 98
yogurt, 88, 131, 174

zinc, 35
zingerone, 63, 103, 146

Penguin Group (USA) Online

What will you be reading tomorrow?

Patricia Cornwell, Nora Roberts, Catherine Coulter,
Ken Follett, John Sandford, Clive Cussler,
Tom Clancy, Laurell K. Hamilton, Charlaine Harris,
J. R. Ward, W.E.B. Griffin, William Gibson,
Robin Cook, Brian Jacques, Stephen King,
Dean Koontz, Eric Jerome Dickey, Terry McMillan,
Sue Monk Kidd, Amy Tan, Jayne Ann Krentz,
Daniel Silva, Kate Jacobs...

You'll find them all at
penguin.com

*Read excerpts and newsletters,
find tour schedules and reading group guides,
and enter contests.*

Subscribe to Penguin Group (USA) newsletters
and get an exclusive inside look
at exciting new titles and the authors you love
long before everyone else does.

PENGUIN GROUP (USA)
penguin.com